Dedication

For my sister, Melissa,
my first and best friend.

Table of Contents

Still The World's Worst Diabetes Mom

MORE REAL-LIFE STORIES OF RAISING A CHILD WITH TYPE 1 DIABETES

Stacey Simms

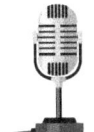

SPARK Publications
Charlotte, North Carolina

Still the World's Worst Diabetes Mom:
More Real-Life Stories of Raising a Child with Type 1 Diabetes
Stacey Simms

Medical Disclaimer:
The information contained in this book is not intended as
medical advice and is not a substitute for the services of and
information from a trained health-care provider.

Designed, produced, and published by SPARK Publications
SPARKpublications.com
Charlotte, North Carolina

Printed in the United States of America
Paperback, October 2022, ISBN: 978-1-953555-36-6
Library of Congress Control Number: 2022917124

❝ My words are meant to help you ask questions of your care team, to have conversations with your child that could benefit your relationship beyond numbers, and, most importantly, to help you realize you're not alone. **❞**

Introduction

I can't believe I'm writing a second book. Some days, I can't believe I wrote the first one. I thought I poured everything I had to say into *The World's Worst Diabetes Mom: Real-Life Stories of Parenting a Child with Type 1 Diabetes.* But after the reactions, emails, and DMs I still get every week, I wanted to say a bit more.

If we haven't met, here's a brief introduction and explanation of "The Worst." My diabetes parenting philosophy is: not perfect, but safe and happy. I was called out on that on social media by another parent who vehemently disagreed. It was a heated exchange and when I gave up arguing, I wrote, "I guess I'm the world's worst diabetes mom."

At that moment, it struck me that everyone did not share my family's feelings about diabetes. We had a positive start in this lousy condition, with an endocrinologist who told us that numbers, while extremely important, shouldn't be allowed to run our lives. He wanted our son, Benny, to grow up as a person with diabetes, not as a person defined by diabetes.

We took our cues from our care team and from thriving families. We realized we were raising a child and not a number or a graph or a lab result. Benny would always be more than his A1C or his Time in Range (TIR).

You don't have to read the first *Worst* to understand and enjoy this book. Of course, I'd love for you to read it as it gives newer diagnosed families of younger children more information about our toddler, preschool, and elementary years.

If you read the first book, you know I only included our experiences up until middle school, basically stopping in sixth grade. Mostly, I felt like I didn't have enough experience with a teen with type 1 diabetes (T1D) and I didn't want to pretend I did. As I write this, Benny is seventeen years old and is about to start his senior year of high school. We're in a much different place now.

Parenting doesn't have a finish line, and we're getting close to college—a completely different phase of diabetes parenting. But I can share, after nearly sixteen years with diabetes, what we've learned and what's worked for us. I'll be the first to tell you: I didn't really expect my teenage Benny to be managing like he does. He really is confident, responsible, and independent, which is what I've tried to teach both of my children, with or without diabetes.

Benny is *far* from perfect. This is not a kid who remembers to pre-bolus for every meal, has nothing but straight continuous glucose monitor (CGM) lines, and changes his infusion set on time exactly every three days.

This *is* a kid who always checks his blood glucose (BG) before driving, manages diabetes independently but will ask for help when he needs it, and talks to friends and coaches about how they can help him thrive with T1D. He's a kid who, without us, went to a country over six thousand miles away at age sixteen and spent this past summer as a Counselor in Training (CIT) at a non-diabetes sleepaway camp.

He's also the kid who left for school the morning I'm writing this and came back five minutes later because his pump was still charging . . . upstairs in his bedroom. Have you seen the needlepoint that says, "World's Okayest Diabetic?" I'm getting that for Benny for his high school graduation.

When I wrote the first book, I was *very* nervous about the reception. As expected, a few people thought I was bananas. They wanted to learn more about how to never spike after eating cereal, how to get their fifteen-year-old to only eat three Skittles for a trending low, and how to dose precisely for pizza. But many others told me about the relief they felt after realizing "safe and happy" was a great goal and that perfection with diabetes isn't an option.

Of course, we're still making all the mistakes, but Benny will be eighteen by the time you're reading this. He's a fully formed human being—no matter what his sister says—and I feel confident our diabetes parenting style has helped him become a happy, healthy, and very independent kid.

This time around, I'm going to continue to share our "world's worst" stories—with all the mistakes I continue to make. I'm also going to shift into offering more been-there parenting advice and quite a few more opinions than last time around. After all this time in the diabetes community, I've seen enough where I feel comfortable letting you know what I think works and what doesn't. But while I think our experiences are helpful, I know our way isn't the only way to manage diabetes.

Diabetes stinks. I don't really know any parents of children with type 1 who think they've got every bit of it right. Are we pushing too much? Are we not doing enough? Will more independence as a teenager mean more complications later? Or will more helicoptering now hurt my relationship with my child and make him resent diabetes even more? Guided by our care team and scientific studies that reassured me that perfection was not the goal, I made my choice long ago. We know Benny can live a long and healthy life even if we aren't flawless with diabetes management.

If you're new here, I don't share Benny's A1C results or any specific numbers unless it's an integral part of the story. I got so many questions about that, I've included an entire chapter about it this time around.

Please don't misunderstand. We take diabetes and Benny's diabetes management and health very seriously. We are vigilant and very involved. I don't keep his numbers out of the public eye because I have something awful to hide. Our endocrinologist is happy about where Benny has spent his childhood in terms of

A1C and is optimistic Benny will be a healthy and happy adult with T1D.

In terms of technology, Benny has used a tubed insulin pump since age two and a half (about six months after diagnosis) and has worn a CGM since 2013—just a few days before he turned nine. We switched to an automated insulin delivery (AID) system in January 2020. It's Tandem's Control-IQ (CIQ), which means he uses a t:slim X2 pump with a Dexcom G6 CGM.

You may wonder how I remember all the stories and details you're about to read. I don't! A few weeks after Benny's diagnosis in 2006, I started writing about our experience with diabetes. I have all those years of blog posts, social media posts, and podcast episode transcripts to use as references.

This is not a book that will tell you how to eat or how to dose. I have no medical degree, nor am I a health care provider. My words are meant to help you ask questions of your care team, have conversations with your child that could benefit your relationship beyond numbers, and, most importantly, to help you realize you're not alone.

I can really sum up our diabetes philosophy in one photo. It's one of Benny, three years old, jumping off our friend's boat into the lake. He's the only one in the photo and he looks like he's ready to leap across the world. He had so much fun that day! He's wearing a life vest and, while you can't see us, there are adults in the boat and in the water. We did what we needed to do to keep Benny safe and happy and then we let him fly.

I show that photo a lot in presentations. Just after I finished the first book, in 2019, I spoke at Friends for Life, an annual family diabetes conference. That's where I met Heather. Her son had been diagnosed for about a year. She was doing great if you go by numbers. Her endocrinologist told her that her son was one of the best-managed kids in their care. But she was terrified. We talked and cried and became fast friends.

After the conference, here's what she wrote on social media:

Thank you FFL. Thank you Stacey Simms . . . . Thank you for teaching me to say yes more, to let go more, to live more. Today it was just me and the T1D at Typhoon Lagoon. Of course he goes straight for the giant wave pool (vicious blood sugar dropping/ Dexcom number hiding pool of death). I hemmed and hawed. He looked at me and said "Mom, sometimes I feel like Nemo and you're Marlin". I remembered all the things I learned this week. I thought about what my new tribe would tell me to do. I vividly remembered Stacey Simms at the closing keynote and the picture of itty-bitty Benny jumping off a boat.

I said yes.

I hated it.

He, of course, lived AND had the time of his life!!!

We decided to celebrate with a giant bucket of ice cream—because now we say yes!!!

Pro tip—no one can tell you are crying at a water park.

Heather is one of many parents who was burdened by the pursuit of perfection, who feared sports or sleepovers, or giant wave pools. I hope this book will help you, like Heather, learn to see that your child can jump off the boat and safely manage those waves.

Your child can fly.

That's a promise from The World's Worst Diabetes Mom.

❝ Forget about the perfect and go for safe and happy. It may amaze you how much your child learns from that philosophy and uses it to thrive along the way. ❞

CHAPTER 1

Am I Secretly the Best?

B efore I tell you about all our mistakes, I want to share one of my proudest parenting moments. Yes, it's a tale that makes me look good! But when it happened, I wasn't even there.

Let's back up and talk a little bit about our family's diabetes story. Benny was diagnosed just before he turned two. In October 2006, he started showing the classic signs you all know. We couldn't keep him in a diaper. He was wetting through multiple times at night and during the day he was sleepy and very thirsty.

For Benny, this would happen a couple of days in a row and then he'd be fine for a week or two. That was just enough for us to keep from calling our doctor. Finally, at Thanksgiving, with other family around and no work or day care, we realized how unusual his behavior was. We called our pediatrician and got a fasting glucose test, which came back at 80 mg/dL, just about perfect. She decided a blood draw was needed and, while horrible at that moment, gave us the gift of an emergency-free and relatively early T1D diagnosis.

In early December 2006, we went to the hospital. Three days later, we came home to start our new life.

At the time, I was working early mornings at my dream job as a morning radio show host and my husband, Slade, owned and operated a restaurant. I left for work at 3:30 a.m. and he was coming home around midnight. We also had a five-year-old daughter, Lea. It was a busy life, but we made it work!

We were incredibly fortunate to bring Benny back to his day care and slowly figured out how to manage diabetes day-to-day.

Slade and I wanted to raise our children to be confident, responsible, and independent—with or without type 1. Yes, we made a ton of mistakes along the way, but I was happy to see Benny making progress, especially as he entered high school.

As a freshman, Benny joined the wrestling team. He's tried all types of sports. I always complain that as soon as we have diabetes and his latest activity figured out, he switches! He played little kid soccer, baseball, and basketball. As he got older, he played middle school football and lacrosse for a quick minute. My favorite, and the one he played the longest, was baseball; a lot of time to manage diabetes in between at-bats! He'd never wrestled before, but tried it anyway.

Like most high school teams around here, there's some traveling involved for the meets. A handful of times during the season, they also stay overnight in hotels when the matches are far away. That was something we never did with my high school sports! We met with Benny's coach very early on to talk about diabetes, mostly as it pertained to practices and matches, and we set out some parameters for these overnight trips.

I also talked to the team mom. She organized fundraisers, helped coordinate the hotel stays, and basically knew everything that was going on. I had contact information for when they were on the road and developed a backup plan.

I'll talk more about our plans for overnights and sleepovers throughout this book. You should know that we remote monitor Benny's Dexcom G6 CGM and we agree on when we'll communicate for what blood sugar numbers. We make a plan for what happens if I can't reach him. For wrestling trips, we agreed I'd call the team mom and then the coach and then the hotel front desk. I also send Benny with more food and low stuff than he'd ever need.

Everything worked out great for the first few trips of the season. But then one night I got an urgent low alert and no response from Benny within our agreed upon time. I waited another fifteen minutes and then texted the team mom. Her son,

Tyler, was in Benny's room that night. They usually have two to three boys in each hotel room—bunkmates rotate every trip.

She texted Tyler, who then told Benny to get back to me. All was well. It was a compression low, which can happen when you lean on the CGM sensor. The circulation in that area slows to a level where the CGM perceives it as low blood sugar. To fix it, all you have to do is simply stop leaning on the sensor. Benny confirmed he felt fine. He just wasn't looking at his phone (obviously). Our system had worked, and I happily went back to bed.

I like to do a debrief on this kind of thing, so when Benny got home, I asked him how he felt about Tyler having to nudge him. It was the first time a friend had to be a sort of diabetes messenger on a wrestling overnight, so I wondered if there was anything he'd prefer I do next time. He said, "No." And then he said this:

"Mom, you really don't have to worry. They all know how to treat an emergency low."

What? How? Turns out, every time Benny was on one of these overnights and in a room with a new set of kids, he would take out his Baqsimi emergency glucagon and explain what it was and how to use it. Baqsimi is a nasal spray. There's no measuring or steps other than opening it up and pressing down. It's easy to use. He would tell the kids that they could use it if they couldn't wake him up or if he was babbling and seemed drunk or didn't make sense. And that they should get the coach, no matter what time of night it was.

Benny said this like it was the most natural thing in the world. He was surprised I didn't realize this was part of his routine.

I always say there's no finish line in parenting, but holy cow, this felt like we had crossed over to a new level! I never specifically asked him to do something like this and yet, he made it a priority. We're lucky Benny has always been comfortable and open about his diabetes, but I hadn't realized how much he was sharing without being asked.

I pushed a little bit further to see what else he was telling the other wrestlers. "I tell everyone I beep overnight. If that's going to bother you, let me know and we'll see if the coach can switch you."

He said no one has ever been bothered. "Mom, no one cares. They usually laugh and say they'll probably snore louder than my beeping." I guess they can sleep through anything at that age.

We are lucky that Benny has never been shy about diabetes, but we didn't get to this level of self-awareness and advocacy overnight. When he was diagnosed, I was terrified to send him back to day care, and I refused to think about anything more than a few days ahead. I had enough trouble just learning to care for my toddler with T1D!

How did we get here? As you'll see in the chapters to come, we had a willingness to try new things, make mistakes, adjust our plans, and keep our sense of humor. We found friends, allies, and helpers along the way.

Like many of you, I was incredibly fearful those first nights in the hospital and the first weeks and months at home. I'm so happy to tell you that none of my fears have come true. I'm superstitious so I hate writing that sentence (someone knock on some wood)! But Benny has had the same opportunities as his sister, Lea, to play sports, travel, spend time with family, go to camp, and so much more. Everyone in our family ate the same food and snacks and treats growing up.

We tried to work diabetes into Benny's life, instead of the other way around. Not prioritizing it 24-7 made some other parents call me out on social media; the "Worst" title is a bit of a joke, but it comes from real criticism and judgment. I shook that off a long time ago, and you should too.

Forget about the perfect and go for safe and happy. It may amaze you how much your child learns from that philosophy and uses it to thrive along the way.

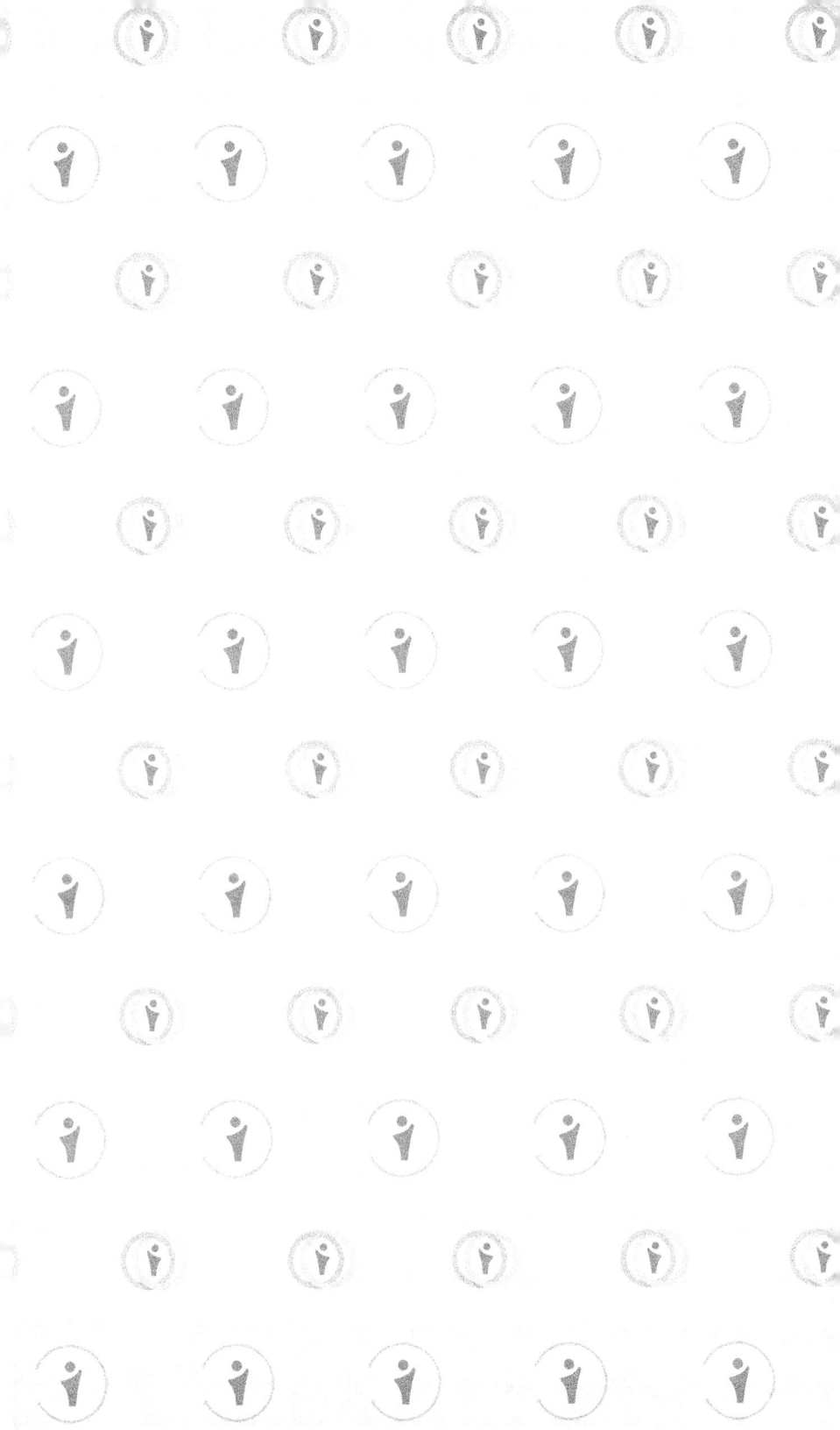

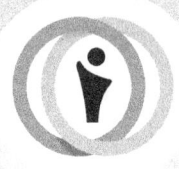

❝ I remember very little about
Benny's blood sugars on Halloween.
But I remember every costume
and I remember all the fun. **❞**

CHAPTER 2

Help for Halloween

There are few holidays that seem scarier to newer diabetes families than Halloween. Candy, running around, costumes that can make diabetes tech difficult to reach, and more candy! Once diabetes is in the picture, it's hard to look at Halloween the same way.

Benny was diagnosed just over a month after Halloween in 2006. When I look back at the photos that year, it's clear something was going on. He was fine one minute and then cranky and tired the next. Of course, we know now that he was in the early stages of type 1. But back then, we were much more concerned with getting the kids' costumes on and heading out with our little red wagon. It's Halloween! Let's go!

That was the only year I got away with dressing the kids as a matched pair. Lea was five and she was Ariel, the Little Mermaid, and Benny, not yet two, was Flounder, Ariel's fish friend. Benny's costume was just a yellow zippy jacket that had Flounder's face as the hood. He loved it and wore it as his actual coat for almost a year after!

As we talk about Halloween strategies, it's important to remember that this has to also feel right for your family. We all parent in our own way, even without diabetes, so why should we expect everyone to "diabetes parent" the same way? That might mean adapting one of the strategies I talk about here, or it may mean coming up with one of your own.

The next Halloween, we had eleven months of diabetes behind us, as well as four months of using an insulin pump. We went to a big Halloween party in our neighborhood where Benny dressed as Bob the Builder. That costume was easy: he wore a plastic hard hat and a tool belt. For trick or treating, he dressed as Rocket from the *Little Einsteins* show, another easy costume. It was pajamas under a ready-made rocket ship rig. It looked sort of like an inner tube with suspenders.

Benny was three years old, and we didn't yet have any kind of CGM. We threw his glucose meter and supplies into his trick or treat bag and headed out. The costumes that year made it easy to reach his insulin pump, so no issues there. It just came down to figuring out what to do with the candy.

Over the years, we tried lots of strategies. Whatever the plan, both kids were allowed to keep a couple of pieces of candy for that night and the next day. We also talked about it in advance, so everyone knew what to expect. A lot of families celebrate Halloween in different ways, and we realized the kids talk about it at school and on the bus. Setting expectations always made it easier.

That first year, Benny traded in all his candy for a toy. I vividly remember it was a Play-Doh—The Backyardigans set. Many people do this now and call it the Switch Witch. We didn't do anything elaborate, like setting out the candy and pretending the Witch came overnight. It was just, hand over the candy and here's your toy! The kids loved it and we did that for maybe two years.

From my blog that first Halloween in 2007:

> Lea was ready to go trick or treating as soon as she came home from school, of course! I convinced her to eat at least a little dinner and she was out the door! She went with friends of ours so Slade could stay home and I could go out with Benny. There was no way Benny could keep up with Lea and her friends. They're like a

pack of wild animals on Halloween . . . actually, more like a pack of golden retriever puppies. Goofy and funny and falling all over each other.

Benny had no interest in getting into his costume or heading out. I was fine with that, but of course it didn't last. As soon as the first group of kids rang our doorbell, the concept of the evening finally clicked. We put on the costume and headed out the door.

Trick or treating with an almost three-year-old is pretty funny. He said "Happy Halloween" to just about everyone we saw and kept offering his candy to other people.

When we got home, I let Benny pick out one piece of candy and then, as we'd discussed, we took the bag away to "trade for a toy!" I decided delayed gratification wasn't the way to go so he got a new Play-Doh set right away. Blood sugar right around 100 all evening long—whoo-hoo!!

Slade bagged up all the candy (I have no idea where it is, I hope he gives it away today) and everyone went to bed. Checked Benny before work this morning at 3:45 a.m. and he was 241. Gave him some insulin and that was it for Halloween. Next stop, Chanukah![1]

A couple of years later, we tried paying for the collected candy. A friend of mine has a child with severe food allergies and this was their method. We decided on a dime for each piece. I almost went with a quarter, but then I remembered how huge Halloween is around here. Good thing—the kids brought home more candy that year than ever! But while the coins were kind of fun, and a bit of a novelty for my digital-era children, money wasn't something that really resonated with them. And who has that many coins on hand?

The next year, my daughter suggested keeping as many pieces of candy as their age. Of course, this was in addition to the stuff we let them eat on Halloween night. I think she heard that from another friend. We talked about it, but I don't remember doing it.

Finally, when Benny was about six or seven, we did Halloween like everyone else. Some candy that night, a few pieces for dessert or a treat over the next week, and then giving whatever's left away to the dentist or another community collection. My kids were always more interested in running all over the neighborhood to collect the candy than in eating a ton of it all at once. Keeping Halloween more "normal" helped make it less stressful for me and I don't think his blood glucose numbers dramatically changed no matter what we did.

Let's talk about the candy itself. I'm sure you've seen the memes and jokes about the after-Halloween "low BG supply" sales. I never thought about keeping the Halloween stash to treat low blood sugars. We had decided early on to only treat lows with juice boxes. There are a couple of reasons for this.

First, I didn't want Benny to think he could only eat candy or dessert when he was low. That's not how our family eats; we enjoy dessert a couple of times a week and we let the kids have sugary snacks here and there. I liked the idea of keeping low treatments boring and uneventful—not something to look forward to. If low treatments were the only time he got a yummy sweet treat, I worried Benny would make himself go low. He's a smart kid. It wasn't an impossible situation to imagine. I didn't want to take that kind of chance.

Second, I also didn't trust myself to not dip into the low supply if it was something I enjoyed. You can shake your head, but I know myself. If there's a giant bag of Halloween candy in my pantry, I'm eating it. So will my husband. And my daughter, without diabetes, will not be happy knowing there's a bag of Snickers or Smarties that's off-limits to her. So, boring juice boxes and peanut butter crackers have stayed as our low-BG treatments even to this day.

If you use candy to treat lows, you should know that not all sweets are created equal for that task. Many people don't realize that different candy affects blood sugar in different ways. There are some terrific carb-counting guides for Halloween, like those from Beyond Type 1 or Project Blue November, but a carb count won't explain the speed of the sugar in these fun-sized candies.

Candy made only with very simple sugar, like dextrose, is going to give you the fastest rise in blood glucose. Skittles, Smarties, and Airheads break down quickly. Chocolate and chocolate-combination treats will bring blood glucose up more slowly. The addition of fat and protein slows down the way the body breaks down glucose. For example, while the combination of chocolate, coconut, and almonds in my beloved Almond Joy is delicious, it will not raise blood glucose as quickly as the simpler candies and it may keep BG elevated for longer periods of time.

It's important to know how candy will influence BG for many reasons, but this one might be unexpected: a lot of kids go low during Halloween, especially overnight. How can that be? Well, after you've done an amazing job of counting and dosing for every carb, your kiddo goes to bed. Most kids walk (or run) around their neighborhoods on Halloween. That's a lot more activity than your child may normally get at 7:00 p.m. on a Tuesday night. It's also exciting, so a lot of kids see their blood sugar shoot up just from adrenaline, a hormone that signals the body to release more glucose and makes them more insulin resistant. If you've treated that, and bolused for every single carb of candy, you'll likely see a big drop a few hours later.

What to do? The first year is always the hardest. Our endo suggested trying to avoid overcorrecting and letting Benny run a little bit higher during trick or treating and at bedtime. Then, not correcting blood glucose for at least three hours after bedtime. That can be hard if you're used to adjusting several times an hour, but sometimes hands-off is the way to go, especially if you're not sure how your child will react.

For us, that meant giving a little bit less insulin at dinner and letting him have two or three pieces of candy without dosing. These days, with newer technology, it could mean setting a temporary basal rate on an insulin pump or putting an AID system into an "exercise" mode. Halloween nights were never perfect, but I can tell you this: we never had an endo appointment where our doctor said, "This is an unhealthy A1C and it's because he went up to 250 on Halloween."

Let's talk about costumes! A tubed pump has always been great for Benny, but it made certain costumes a bit more challenging. Have you ever tried to dig out an insulin pump from under an Iron Man body suit? I hear you Omnipod people and yes, this is one of those times when the remote control is a tremendous help. But we always got it done.

It never occurred to me to plan Benny's costume around his pump access; that just doesn't seem fair. Most children don't care if there's a little bulge somewhere under their costume. They just want to dress up and have fun. Please don't worry about getting to the pump every second, or what the gear looks like to you. Just let him pretend he's Iron Man!

When Benny was young enough that one of us would go door-to-door with him, I probably checked his blood glucose on every corner. As we grew more comfortable, we only checked if he said he felt off or started acting wonky. After all, if he was low, we had tons of sugar right there with us!

As he got older and wanted to run around with friends, Benny had the same rules as his older sister without diabetes: check in with us every hour (they were almost always back at our house more often to guzzle some water or take off part of their costume because it was hot) and don't go too far from the house. We live in a huge neighborhood, so they had a sizeable area to roam, but we wanted them to stay within a few blocks. Once Benny had a CGM, it got a little easier, but we never really changed up the routine. As an older teen, Benny now just hangs out with friends and watches horror movies or he stays home and gives out the candy!

We had a big milestone around Halloween one year. When he was ten, Benny decided to take a pump break in October. After eight years of wearing an insulin pump, he said he was tired of the infusion set changes and wanted a break. I was not happy, but I supported his decision. We'd always said that it didn't matter how insulin got into his body, as long as he made sure that it did.

I told him I would not give him shots; he'd have to do that himself. I spoke about this in the first book. It may be hard to believe, but many kids who go on insulin pumps when they're very young grow up just as scared of shots as kids who never had them! At age two, Benny was up to eight shots a day and he didn't care one bit. But by age ten, he didn't remember any of that and he was terrified.

Letting him take a pump break turned out to be the way to get him over his fear of giving himself injections. We talked about what a break would really look like. Would I follow him to school and to friends' homes to give him shots? Would I meet him on his bike down the block if he stopped for a snack? He realized quickly that he did not want his mom around that much, so he'd have to do it himself. We sat together for about twenty minutes before he worked up enough courage to give himself the first shot. It was a huge milestone for him!

As proud as we all were, that pump break didn't last very long. Halloween itself was fine, but Benny went very low overnight. We hadn't really figured out the long-acting dose and we realized the more precise basal dosing of a pump can be very helpful. For the next couple of days, he wanted to eat a little more after a meal, but that meant taking another shot. He decided on his own that he preferred the pump and put it back on after about four days.

We got an interesting question on my podcast, *Diabetes Connections*, about Halloween. My friend, Moira McCarthy, is a long-time diabetes advocate and author. She and I have *Ask the D-Moms* episodes where we answer listeners' questions. This question was from a mom who said her child was newly diagnosed and the child didn't want to celebrate Halloween that year. How could she encourage her daughter to get back out there and enjoy what she had previously loved?

Moira and I asked whether she liked Halloween in the past? If so, maybe just push her a little to have fun and go with her friends for a couple of blocks, depending on age. You can reassure your child that you'll be the diabetes fixer that night. You can worry about carb counting and dosing so the child can just have fun.

If Halloween isn't a big deal, or she is too nervous to even try, maybe have her dress up and answer the door. That was Moira's suggestion and I think it's great. My kids loved doing that when they were in that tween age when they felt a little old for trick or treating but still too young for parties. If they're really into the holiday, you can make your house the one with a theme or where there are activities on the lawn or front porch for younger kids. The idea is to just make sure the child knows diabetes isn't the end of all fun.

If a child fears what might happen if she goes low while walking around or too high from candy, I'd encourage her to share those fears. Talk it out and reassure her; thousands of kids with diabetes have managed this holiday before. If you're not sure what to say, this might be a good time to have your care team talk to her. Sometimes it can be more reassuring coming from the doctor, especially for older tweens or teens who seem to listen to anyone other than their mom!

A quick note about well-meaning neighbors. That first year, a lot of wonderful people in our neighborhood tried to give Benny the sugar-free candy they had bought especially for him. So thoughtful, so nice, and so unnecessary. Also, not great for your stomach (you can go google more about that, but I'm warning you, it's gross). Luckily, I had been warned about the potential for bathroom issues, so I separated and removed the sugar-free candy before anyone could eat it.

We also had a neighbor who tried really hard but missed the mark. She was so happy to see us! "Wait right here," she said.

"I have something special for you." We waited a few moments, looking at the giant bowl of Milk Duds and Airheads she was giving to the other trick or treaters. She came back and very proudly handed a special pencil to Benny.

He was not happy with the pencil. But he knew to be respectful and polite. We thanked everyone and took the pencil, just as we had done with the sugar-free candy. The following year, I did a little preemptive work at the bus stop. I started saying things like, "We've learned so much about diabetes this year. It turns out that sugar-free candy is really not good for Benny. And our doctor says we can just do a normal Halloween, so please give him what you're giving everyone else!" It worked out very well and there were no more pencils collected that year, or any year since!

It's very common to feel like life after diabetes will never be the same; holidays like Halloween really nail that point home. But most diabetes families find a way through with a new routine that works for them. In the long run, I remember very little about Benny's blood sugars on Halloween. But I remember every costume and I remember all the fun.

ASK YOUR DOCTOR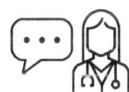

- Knowing my child's age and stage of diabetes, what should we adjust for Halloween? Should we change any dosing?

- Have you heard of any creative ideas from our local community about how they manage Halloween?

- Do you have a carb count for Halloween candy?

" Will you worry? Of course! I still do! We can't let that stop our kids from developing confidence and self-reliance. Small steps now will help them build to a more independent future. **"**

CHAPTER 3

Sleepovers

My daughter, Lea, told me something interesting after her first month at college. She said the first few weeks of freshman year, you could tell who had never been away from home. The kids who hadn't been on school overnights or away to camp, she said, had a much harder time adjusting.

My daughter's opinion is hardly a medical study, but that rings true to me. Looking back, starting small with sleepovers with grandparents, then with friends, then time away at camp helped us build on what we learned and gradually become more comfortable. What can seem to us like a scary night away from home can also be looked at as a building block to future independence.

In terms of building blocks, let me share where we are right now. As I write this chapter, Denny is just home from a weekend away. He's going to be a Counselor in Training (CIT) at his non-diabetes camp this summer; this was a team building weekend for that group.

We had no conversations with staff, other than filling out the usual forms and noting that he has type 1. I didn't text him about blood sugars, although I could see he went a little low the first night and very high after breakfast the second day (it was an obvious late bolus; he came down a little while later). I helped with prep and packing because, at this stage, that's part of our agreement. For now, I still check the diabetes bag. We also talked about what kind of low stuff to take. I don't think we texted or talked the entire time he was gone.

This is *not* the way I handled sleepovers or nights away when Benny was younger. Our actions back then have led to being more hands-off now. Of course, we messed up a lot along the way.

Before I jump in, let's acknowledge that not everyone likes sleepovers, with or without diabetes. Is it terrible to admit I hate them? No one sleeps and if they're younger, somebody always wants to go home in the middle of the night. There's a lot of eating and it's a noisy mess. If they're too quiet, then you know trouble's brewing. We've hosted our share and we've let our kids go to bunches, but it doesn't mean I'm a fan.

If your rule is no sleepovers, or none until a certain age, just make sure that's a "family" rule and not a "diabetes" rule. Kids keep track of this stuff and we have found it very helpful to create family rules rather than diabetes-specific ones whenever possible.

We settled on age seven for our kids. That's common around our neighborhood, with most children that age in first or second grade. Lea was invited to a few in kindergarten, but we thought that was just too young. For those, we'd pick her up around 10:00 p.m. and sometimes bring her back if there was a fun breakfast the next day.

With Benny, we settled on the same age, but knew we needed to do some more work. We decided Benny would, with supervision, check his own blood glucose and give his own insulin. He'd been doing that since kindergarten, so it wasn't as big a deal as it might be for some seven-year-olds.

My friends were all very comfortable supervising and helping Benny with his diabetes care. They seemed less comfortable doing fingersticks and giving injections. Pressing buttons on the pump or pump remote would be easy, but again, Benny did that early on. You may have a relationship with your friends where they take care of everything diabetes related. We did not. And that didn't stop us.

There really is nothing wrong with giving your child a goal to be a bit more self-sufficient. "If you want to go on sleepovers, let's work on doing these things." It's often the way a lot of kids step up to doing diabetes tasks they don't normally do.

Interestingly, even though Benny was basically independent by early elementary school (again, with supervision) he always leaned on us heavily at home. That was fine with me; it's a lot to ask a young child to be completely independent and most health professionals advise against it. While he did his own fingersticks at school and at his friends' homes, at our house, we still did almost all of his care until well into middle school.

At age seven, Benny didn't have a continuous glucose monitor (CGM). He started with a CGM at age nine, but the Share and Follow functions, which allow a caregiver to see blood glucose numbers remotely, wasn't available until he was closer to eleven. Is life better with it? Heck yeah! Would I give it back? No, I would not. But it's important to realize you can be safe and have fun without a CGM. I hate when I hear parents pull kids from activities and sleepovers because the Dexcom isn't working.

Before we had a CGM, we'd check in with Benny at dinner and before bed. He didn't have a cell phone, so we'd text or call the parent. At the dinner check, we'd talk about what his BG was at the moment, where it had been at the previous checks, what he was eating, whatever activity was about to happen, and then we'd make a plan.

The activity was always the trickiest. Sometimes they'd be playing outside for hours after dinner, but sometimes they'd just sit and watch a movie. Knowing how active he'd be helped us figure out the dosing. Our usual plan was to give a lot less fast-acting insulin for dinner. Then I'd call or text back around 10:00 or 11:00 p.m. and we'd evaluate and move on to the plan for the rest of the night.

It's funny to look back at these stories from our current time, when everyone's kid seems to have a cell phone, even if it's just for remote monitoring. Benny didn't have one until fifth grade and he didn't even carry it with him until middle school. I feel like a Stone Age parent! Using a CGM and cell phone to share blood glucose numbers remotely is a game changer, mostly because you can get a much fuller picture of what's happening, rather than relying on one moment in time. But again, you can do it all safely, if not quite as precisely, with older technology.

Usually, our routine and decision-making leaned on giving a little less insulin and running Benny a little higher overnight during nights away. Ask your doctor about this. We always bumped up the target range. That can mean extra math with multiple daily injections, or some pump setting changes. If you use one of the newer AID systems, it may be as easy as switching to a different target (if that's an option) or to an "exercise" mode. You could also create a basal profile called "sleepover" that gives less insulin overall. Whatever the insulin delivery method, we wanted the result to be a higher BG target during this one night.

I can hear you yelling at me, "I don't want to increase my child's target range! We keep it tight at eighty-five!" If that's the case, you might have a problem with sleepovers. I certainly don't think the first one is the time to worry about supertight control; you'll be setting yourself—and your child—up for a lot of stress.

To be clear, I'm not talking about going wild and cranking the target up to 300. If your target range is 80–120, move it to 120–200 for the night. If, like us, it's more 80–180, bump it to 150–220. This is an endo-type question, so ask what they might recommend.

Remember, setting a target BG doesn't mean that's what will actually happen! Even with the newer AID systems, a lot of factors go into where BG lands. The idea here is to avoid extremes and lessen stress. For us, even moving the target higher meant that Benny would usually end up lower all night. But he'd be safely lower, closer to 100 or 120 rather than tanking down to 55.

If your child is on multiple daily injections (MDI), what about adjusting long-acting? Depending on what kind you use, it can take more than a day to see any changes, so this isn't usually recommended. Most moms I know will just give that long-acting shot a little earlier than usual for that one day so the child doesn't have to worry about it at the sleepover. This is another great question for the care team.

I'd also make a plan for lows—something beyond, "I'm sure they have juice in the fridge." I always send low stuff with Benny; I never assume that someone has what he'll need. And even if their house is stocked with treats and sugary drinks, your child might not have easy access at 2:00 a.m. when the Dexcom is going off.

For example, Benny had a friend who had a fridge in the garage full of different flavored sodas. I've never seen anything like it: glass bottles, wild flavors, fun stuff. But if his blood sugar went low at 3:00 a.m., would I want Benny to make his way from the kids' second-floor bedroom all the way to the garage? Not a great idea.

This family also had a pool and Benny later told me he drank two of the sodas with no bolusing. Apparently, there was a lot of late-night swimming! I told you that activity is bananas.

We usually sent Benny with a medium-sized bottle of Gatorade. I think it's about 25–30 carbs. That's a lot more than I'd give for a regular overnight low, but it made it easy on him. Our rule on sleepovers was, if you wake up and feel wonky, drink at least some of the Gatorade first, then check your blood sugar. Before the CGM, it was drink then fingerstick, then it was drink, then look at your receiver. I'm pretty sure these days he checks his phone first, but I still stand by the idea that if you feel low, better to get some quick sugar in you before you rely on your brain to make decisions. This has worked very well for us; he's never downed the Gatorade when he didn't really need it. And if he did, I'd prefer that! He can always correct a high.

Most kids are shyer than we may think at someone else's house. They may feel weird about leaving the bedroom where everyone is finally asleep to sneak out to the kitchen. It's a strange house and they don't want to wake people up. This is important to talk about, because most kids are polite and they feel rude about waking people up, even if they need help.

We had to drive that message home after we realized Benny didn't understand. About five years ago, we spent an overnight away on our anniversary. It wasn't far, less than an hour, but the kids were only fifteen and twelve, so we got a sitter. While we were out, Benny and the sitter called and asked if he could sleep over at his friend's house, just behind ours. Sure, no problem, sounds like fun. We made sure he had what he needed in his diabetes bag, and he walked over.

Here's my Facebook post about what happened overnight:

> OMG . . . all is well . . . blood sugars were fine overnight. However, he decided to come home around 4:30 a.m. He told his friend, called our sitter and walked home (our backyards are connected and she waited for him outside). BUT they never told the host parents. We had a long talk this morning with both boys about why that might have been important, especially because Benny decided to come home because his BG was on the low side (76) and he didn't want to bother them for juice. Seriously?! This is not our first rodeo. The sitter didn't call us because she assumed the host parents knew and there was no need to get us involved. So we had a really nice (and clueless) night away! ☺

Let's talk about what you're doing at home during all this. If you remote monitor, you might think, 'Well, that's easy. I'll just stay up and watch the numbers all night long.' You could do that, but I'd urge you to think it through and make a plan.

Ask yourself, when would you call your child or the other parent? When do you need to intervene? This is a personal decision you'll make based on your child's age, experience, and expertise. When Benny was eight, my plan for this looked very different from the plan I mentioned at the start of this chapter!

This is a time to sit down with your child and talk about expectations. Benny knows if he stays under a certain number for a certain amount of time, I'm going to check on him. Same thing with a higher number. Again, this has changed a lot over time, but we still know the parameters. You can then share this with the host parent.

I think this is where it gets a bit tricky. It's that fine line of not wanting to scare people. We don't want our children excluded because diabetes is too much work. But realistically, there are some things other parents need to know. I don't think there's anything wrong with asking the host parent to keep their phone off of silent mode for the night. I always say, if I know I can call you, I'll sleep. And you can call me with any questions as well.

For us, remote monitoring at sleepovers had a bit of a rough start. Quick history: the Dexcom Share system as we know it today—transmitter directly to phone or medical device via Bluetooth—was approved in late 2015 and adopted by most users in 2016. Prior to that, the data went from the transmitter to the receiver via radio frequency, and then to the phone using Bluetooth. And, for a very brief time, you had to use something called the Dexcom Share Cradle.

It sounds bonkers now, but you would take the Dexcom receiver and slip it into a larger standing base. It cradled the receiver and the two parts connected via a tiny USB port. Once connected, the cradle would use Bluetooth to send the data to a smartphone.

We had that cradle, and I thought it worked well at home. But taking it anywhere was a bit of a challenge. It wasn't meant to be portable, and it had a hard time connecting; you sort of had to find the perfect spot for it to work. Even so, I know people who plugged it into a battery pack and threw it in their backpack.

We took it to exactly one sleepover. This was at one of my best friends' homes. Karen has known us since shortly after

Benny's diagnosis, so she's always up for trying diabetes stuff. We spent at least fifteen minutes trying to figure out where to put the cradle. We had to find a place where it picked up the Wi-Fi and where it would still pick up Benny as he slept. Finally, we decided on a spot, and I left for the night. Twenty minutes after I drove away, Karen called to let me know Benny's Dexcom sensor had come out. Of course. I told her to forget the whole thing and just tell him to fingerstick as usual. So I guess we never really used the cradle at any sleepover!

As I said, the next cradle-free iteration was approved less than a year later. Still, it's worth noting that Dexcom Share, in any form, has been around only since 2014. The amazing Do-It-Yourself diabetes community figured it out a bit earlier than that. The first DIY sharing I know of was reported in 2013.

Even with the modern—and much easier—Share and Follow apps, if your child is younger, let's say still in elementary school, I highly recommend a sleepover test run. I loved doing this with newer friends, even into middle school. It was almost an overnighter; Benny would go over for dinner and then hang out until 10:00 or 11:00 p.m. That way, Benny could eat and stay long enough for the new friends to get a good idea of what diabetes is about.

I recommend sending emergency glucagon on sleepovers. You have three relatively easy options to choose from: Baqsimi is a nasal spray, Gvoke and Zegalogue are pre-mixed auto injectors. Check with your endo and insurance to see which option may be best. Some people just prefer to send cake icing, which works well. Consider cutting off the tip and putting the tube in a plastic bag. If you've ever used tubed cake icing, you know getting that tip off can be difficult and you don't want to struggle with it during an emergency!

When I talk to other parents about this, I always say that in sixteen years of diabetes, we've never had to use glucagon. But that's not true for everyone. And while it can seem scary to explain why it might be needed, in my opinion, it's scarier to leave the host parents ignorant, especially if your child is young enough that their friends may not understand what to do for a severe low.

When you host a sleepover, you're taking on an enormous responsibility. It's not just about our kids with diabetes. The parents have to be prepared if something happens to any kid in their house.

When I was about eight years old, I had a sleepover and my friend cut her leg on the edge of my trundle bed. This was in the 1970s, so of course the bed was metal. That cut was bad; it was deep enough that we had to go to the hospital! My parents weren't even there; the sitter had to take all of us to the emergency room where my friend got stitches. I think about that a lot; with or without diabetes, the host parents must be prepared for minor issues and more serious situations. A child can choke on a piece of food, have a low blood sugar, or cut their leg deeply enough to need stitches.

This has helped me explain diabetes to other parents. For us, a T1D emergency is extremely rare and it's been helpful to frame it that way. However, if you've used glucagon several times, your child goes very low (under 55) more often, or has another underlying medical condition, it's a good idea to talk to your endo before a sleepover. There may be other factors to keep in mind.

It's an awful lot to think about, but most families with T1D manage to figure out how to make sleepovers fun and safe. And it gets easier as they get older. By the time Benny reached high school, our check-ins for sleepovers changed dramatically. Now I'll text him around 10:00 or 11:00 p.m. and just ask, "You good?"

What that means is: "Do you have low stuff? Is your insulin pump charged and full of enough insulin to get you through the night? Is Dexcom behaving, and are you sure the sensor session isn't about to end? And, besides diabetes, is everything OK at your friend's house?"

That little shorthand comes out of discussions with Benny over the years. It's a compromise between what he needs to have fun and not feel like I'm nagging or hovering and my need for him to stay safe. Remember, we didn't start out with that shorthand. It comes from years of experience, lots of Gatorade and texting, and a few mistakes—like that jaunt across my neighbor's lawn!

I think the bottom line with sleepovers is that they are a fun way to start your kid thinking about independence. They are truly not the time to worry about a supertight blood sugar range. There's going to be weird food and unusual activity, but you can find ways to make it fun and safe. Will you worry? Of course! I still do! That's just being a parent. We can't let our worry stop our kids from developing confidence and self-reliance. Small steps now will help them build to a more independent future.

ASK YOUR DOCTOR

■ Do you think my child is ready for sleepovers?

■ Is there a different target range you'd recommend for sleepovers and, if so, what kinds of insulin dosing adjustments would you recommend?

■ If we don't already have one, would you prescribe a newer type of easy-to-use glucagon, such as the nasal spray or an auto-injector?

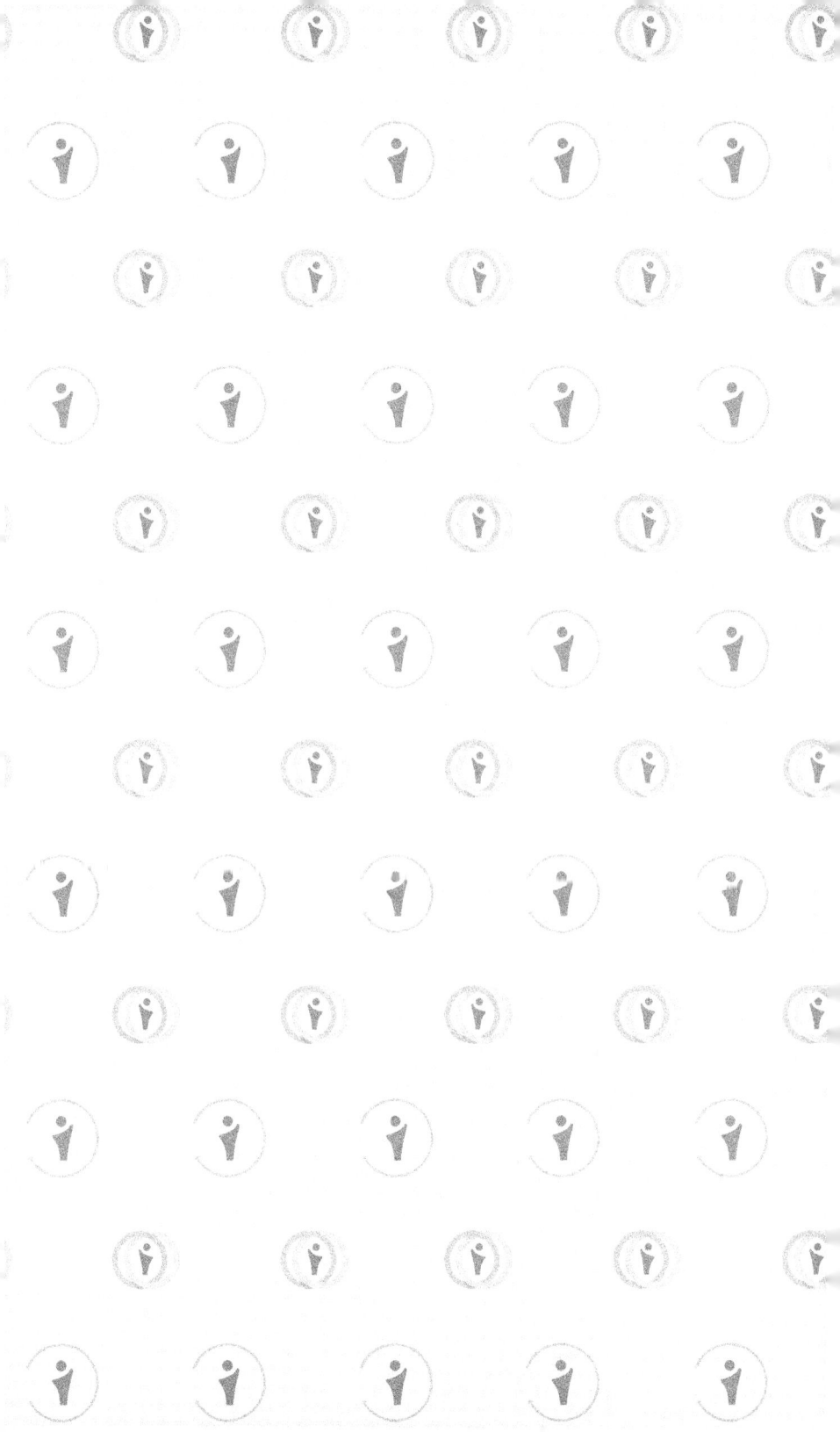

❝ What is Benny's sugar usually
like from 1:45 to 3:05 p.m.?" I
resisted the urge to email back,
"Depends on whether Mercury
is in retrograde that day. **❞**

CHAPTER 4

School Days

I got a call yesterday from the high school nurse. It's the end of the school year and she asked if Benny could stop by and get his supplies out of her office. "Of course," I said. "He'll come by after his last final today." When I hung up, I realized it's only the second time I've had a conversation with her all year and the first was when her refrigerator broke. How did we get from fearfully sending him to kindergarten to barely thinking about diabetes during the school day?

I spent a lot of time in the first book talking about school; I won't rehash everything here. But since that book ended just as middle school was starting, there's more to share. Benny needed a very different routine in the toddler room at day care than he did in elementary school, middle school, and now finishing up high school.

We've always stressed communication and over the years, I've done a lot of emailing with Benny's teachers. We've been lucky to have a lot of support and understanding from school staff. But it's difficult to explain all the ins and outs of type 1 diabetes. In middle school, one teacher wanted to make sure her class time was covered. She asked me, "What is Benny's sugar usually like from 1:45 to 3:05 p.m.?" I resisted the urge to email back, "Depends on whether Mercury is in retrograde that day."

In terms of care, Benny has been almost completely independent since the end of fifth grade. Starting in kindergarten, he always tested and treated in class, only going to the nurse for extra supplies or if he didn't feel well. We carried that into middle school.

At the time, he was using the Animas insulin pump (no longer in production) and the Dexcom CGM. He switched to the Tandem t:slim X2 by eighth grade, but neither system was automated. Benny was responsible for all the checking, dosing, and correcting while at school.

We stayed in the same school district, so the move to middle school just took a quick meeting to update our 504 plan. This plan refers to Section 504 of the 1973 Rehabilitation Act. It's there to make sure any child with a disability at a public school receives accommodations that will provide support and remove barriers. You may have also heard of an Individualized Education Program (IEP), which is a bit different. An IEP provides more individualized special education and often requires more documentation. These are very simplified explanations of rather complex documents, so please check with your school and your doctor to decide what your child needs.

In our district, we also have something called a Diabetes Care Plan (DCP). This lays out pretty much everything about how the child manages T1D; it's signed by your doctor and contains a lot of information that might be in other children's 504 plans. I mention it here because our experience with the 504 plan was only for graded testing. We had those accommodations in place since third grade and had learned what Benny really needed and wanted.

Simply, Benny may keep his technology on, even if it beeps, and be able to stop testing time for bathroom breaks and water as needed. He was not to take a test if his BG was under 85 or above 250. These accommodations were for major tests, but Benny knew he could always speak up if he needed additional help in school. Some 504 plans and DCPs are much more detailed; it's important to tailor the plans around your child's needs.

Because Benny's insulin pump displays his Dexcom value, there was no need to keep his phone in his pocket or on his desk during testing. Most of the classrooms in our school now have little cubbies where the kids place their phones, so they're not tempted to use them during class. Benny either put his phone in there or gave it to the teacher or proctor. I rarely remote monitored during testing, but in middle school, we kept it as an option.

Our beginning-of-school communication changed completely in sixth grade. In elementary school, I'd have an in-person meeting, usually with the nurse, the teacher, and either the principal or the school counselor. We'd go over all the information, Benny's DCP and 504 plan. We'd look at the class schedule and figure out how to fit BG checks and dosing into the day. I'd also explain about the ups and downs of diabetes, show them the technology and, when Benny was younger, donate a diabetes book to the classroom. We'd talk about letting Benny eat whatever birthday treats or special snacks came into school and how to deal with more active gym or field days.

In sixth grade, I still met with the nurse just before school started. But that was it! Other than the 504 meeting with the school counselor, I didn't meet any of the staff until the open house night a few weeks later. That felt incomplete to me; I wanted to set Benny up for success and let the teachers know I was happy to be involved. I decided to email his team all at once. I wasn't exactly sure how much to say. Here's what I settled on, which mentions the new watch we were trying out:

Hello teachers!

My son, Benny, is one of your students this year.

Benny has type 1 diabetes and I wanted to send this email so we're all on the same page.

Of course, we're already working with (the school nurse) and she is cc'd on this email.

Benny was diagnosed with type 1 just before he turned two, so this is not a new situation.

He wears an insulin pump and a continuous glucose monitor (CGM).

Benny is responsible for his own diabetes care.

He will check blood sugar and administer insulin as needed.

Benny's CGM (called a Dexcom) sends his blood glucose values to his phone and then to a watch he wears.

I will check in with Benny once a day via text message to the watch.

He will text back to me, likely during lunch or in the hallway.

Benny is very wary of extra attention and does not want to disrupt class.

If it becomes a distraction in any way, please let me know.

This is our first year using the watch and I expect to modify as we go.

He will keep his phone in his string bag on silent. The watch should be set to vibrate.

On days when Benny isn't wearing the CGM, he will use a blood sugar meter to test.

Benny will carry other diabetes supplies in his string bag and knows to treat low and high blood sugars.

If he becomes so low that he is disoriented, dizzy or shaky, please send him to the nurse along with another student.

Please email or call with any questions.

Benny is usually very happy to answer questions about diabetes, but I'm not sure he'll want to address it too much the first few days. You all have much more experience with middle-schoolers than I do and I'm sure you'll handle this situation in a way that makes everyone comfortable.

Thanks! Looking forward to a great year.

Best,

Stacey

Too much? Not enough? Can you tell I'm that nervous middle school mom, trying to figure out where the line is between pushing independence and not wanting to let go?

Most of the teachers emailed back to just say thanks for the heads up. But this is the email that prompted one teacher to ask about his BG specifically during the time of her class. I wish I could have reassured her that he'd be perfect from 1:45 to 3:05 p.m.!

You can see from that email we had started using a smartwatch. It was a Pebble Watch and that was our one use of DIY technology. It was such a great little system. Benny could see his BG and we could text back and forth using the watch. That once-a-day text that I mentioned earlier was something we agreed on. I would text him every day about ten minutes before lunch with a reminder to bolus. If nothing wacky was going on, that would be our only communication during the school day.

I tried to text Benny as little as possible while at school. Honestly, it was very difficult for me to restrain myself. Middle school was rough on diabetes management.

Like a lot of kids, Benny was a diabetes superstar early on but got less interested in advocacy and talking about it as he got older. I think there's sort of a diabetes "golden age" between five and ten. These kids want to cut the ribbon at the JDRF Walk, showoff their technology, and talk to just about anyone about T1D. By age ten or eleven, they often become more reluctant and withdrawn, not necessarily rebelling or slacking off, but a bit more self-conscious and unwilling to make diabetes the center of attention. It's completely age-appropriate, according to most parenting experts I've asked. Most kids come back to themselves in their later teen years and many young adults with T1D are incredible advocates.

When middle school started, Benny was very independent with his care, but what I call "brain fog" had set in. Middle school is such a hard time, with or without diabetes. I don't need to tell you that puberty is rough all around. Your body is going bananas. You're in a new school with more responsibility, and you just want to fit in. I thought I'd be dealing with burnout or rebellion. Instead, I had a kid who still seemed to care about his diabetes and wanted to be responsible, but who kept forgetting things that seemed easy to remember just a few months before.

I think I'm lucky, though, because we'd been through this before with his older sister who doesn't have diabetes. Some things are just regular old tween and teen issues; it's not all about T1D.

By the end of the eighth grade, it seemed like Benny's brain had landed back inside his head. We had switched to an untethered method that year as well, and his diabetes management and mindset had really improved. (I'll talk more about that in chapter 11.) It wasn't all smooth sailing, but he was increasingly independent while staying in a healthier range.

Later, while we were discussing high school, he thanked me for not getting on his case more in middle school. I asked him to share more about what he meant, and he confided that there was another student he'd seen at the nurse's office who was often very low. Benny said the boy was making himself go low on purpose—giving too much insulin—because his parents had promised him an expensive video game system if he could keep his A1C down. I understand those parents' fears and wanting to keep their son safe and healthy, but that's a tough way to go about it. Rewarding on the numbers, instead of on the management, can be tricky. Our kids are smart, but they don't always think things through. That boy missed a lot of class and could have really hurt himself trying to please his well-meaning parents.

The beginning of high school was like an abbreviated version of our entry into middle school. We had a quick talk with the nurse to drop off supplies, reviewed the 504 plan with the counselor, and emailed his teachers. As you'll see, it was a little shorter than the previous email and mostly about technology:

Hi all!

As we get closer to the first day of school, I wanted to send a quick note about my son, Benny.

Benny has type 1 diabetes.

There's really nothing special you need to know except that he carries a cell phone and wears an Apple Watch as part of his medical care.

The watch displays his blood sugar number and we occasionally use it to text about diabetes if needed.

This is all laid out in the Diabetes Care Plan and 504 plan.

Benny knows not to use his phone/watch for any other purpose during school and we have not had an issue.

He also wears an insulin pump and uses a continuous glucose monitor—so he may beep every now and then.

Benny is meeting with the nurse tomorrow and he knows to see her with any issues. All we ask is that you excuse him if he indicates he needs to see the nurse and that he be allowed to use the bathroom at any time (high blood sugars increase the need to urinate. Benny is very well controlled, but type 1 diabetes is unpredictable).

I know Benny won't see every teacher on this list first semester, but I thought it would be easier to email everyone now. Thank you so much!

Best,

Stacey.

I'm sure it thrilled everyone that I talked about peeing in my back-to-school email! As you know, that's an important aspect of diabetes. But please don't tell Benny I wrote about it!

He went to a big public high school—there were over 600 kids in his ninth-grade class and the nurse told us there were twenty-one students with type 1 in the school. The staff was supportive, but it wasn't something that anyone seemed surprised or worried about.

Our 504 meeting wasn't very eventful, but we talked about why it was important to have this plan in place for high school. College admission exams like the SAT and ACT will allow for accommodations, but it's not a fast process and they often rely on the school for information. We could use Benny's 504 plan for both tests, but the ACT test process also asked for some sort of proof he has type 1 diabetes! I thought that was silly, but our endocrinologist knew what to provide. If your child hasn't had a 504 at all, ninth grade is a good time to ask for one, if just to get ready for the college boards.

During Benny's freshman year, he asked me to continue to text him before lunch. I was surprised, but he said, "If you can help me with diabetes stuff, I can just concentrate on school stuff." That made sense to me, and I was more than happy to help! I would continue to text "lunch bolus" until he told me to stop. To be clear, he *still* didn't always remember to do it. But my texting was helpful overall.

We had great support from the staff, but we also had a handful of times where someone was reluctant to give Benny the benefit of the doubt and went against what was in our 504 plan. I told Benny that we would always have his back when it came to diabetes at school. If he was low and needed to treat when no one else was allowed food, or if he had to go to the bathroom when it wasn't the "right" time, he should just do what he needed. If he got in trouble, we'd get him out of it. My kids are both real rule-followers and this was a hard concept, especially in middle school.

Benny understood what I meant when, one year, he told his teacher he was getting a migraine. I don't talk about this a lot, but he would get frequent migraines in elementary and into middle school. We tried to eliminate as many triggers as we could find, and he seems to have outgrown them (knock on wood), but at the time, the migraines were brutal. Benny told his fourth-grade teacher he could feel one coming on and she told him to sit back down. After trying to cope with the beginnings of a migraine, he finally puked in her classroom. She believed him after that.

You hope your kid never has to go against what a teacher or school staff member says, but I think it's worth a quick conversation, so they know you're in their corner. For us, this was only for health care reasons; I will not plead his case if he's rude or doesn't follow "regular" rules. The migraine story helped Benny understand what I was talking about; going forward he would just get up and go to the nurse when he felt one coming on. The nurse would call his teacher and explain.

Freshman year in high school for Benny was also freshman year in college for my daughter. There was a lot going on, but we transitioned relatively smoothly. Lea was settled and enjoying her first year away, and Benny jumped into high school with enthusiasm. Diabetes was behaving relatively well. That's when everything changed, and not just for us.

This was the 2019–2020 school year, so you can probably see what I'm getting at. COVID-19 closed Benny's high school in mid-March and Lea came home from college right around the same time. My daughter returned to college that fall—her school did a fabulous job with masking, testing, and isolating; and they had almost all classes in person after August 2020. Benny, though, spent his sophomore year of high school at home with remote learning.

Honestly, diabetes was relatively easy to manage during this time. There were several reasons for that. At the end of eighth grade, Benny's interest in fitness increased and he started working out more. He grew quite a few inches, gained a lot of muscle, and started thinking more about what he was eating. We also switched to Control-IQ in January 2020 and immediately saw the benefits of an AID system. All of that together meant the lowest A1Cs we'd ever seen, with less work than we'd ever done. It was wild!

Benny went back to in-person class in August 2021. He's finishing up that junior year as I'm writing this book. It's been a tough year academically and I think the adjustment back to in-person classes was difficult as well, at least for a few weeks.

I've had to adjust too. I no longer text before lunch and I only get involved if I think he's really got an issue.

Which brings us to that message from the nurse. There have been high and low blood sugar levels this year, of course. And Benny has occasionally called me to bring him a cartridge of insulin and even a charger for his pump once. But I can count the number of times he's called about diabetes this year on one hand. It's been surprisingly uneventful, especially as I think back to middle school!

I mentioned we stressed communication with staff over the years. I also focused very much on communication with Benny. Every year we sit down and have a conversation about how he wants school to go that year. Does he have new goals? Challenges he wants help to face? In first grade, a goal could be buying a school lunch once a week instead of always bringing lunch from home. In eleventh grade, it was managing all diabetes care by himself during the school day, with no input or texts from me unless it was an agreed-upon dangerous situation.

I love these talks. You can learn a lot about what your children are thinking about by asking them what they want to accomplish. Yes, as Benny got older, the conversations were often met with eye rolls and heavy sighs. But all this time, he's known that we value his input and we listen to him. I think it's made a big difference in his confidence and independence.

Even so, I am frankly amazed that my former sixth grader with brain fog spent his junior year waking himself up for school and getting out the door every morning with no help from me. I feel like I blinked and the twelve-year-old who needed me to find his socks is now a rising senior who rarely asks for my help. I'm grateful that he knows I'm here if he needs it. He's on his own with the socks!

ASK YOUR DOCTOR

- Our child is moving to middle or high school. What questions would you recommend we ask the school?

- Do you have any examples of 504 or Diabetes Care Plans we can use to get ours started?

- Are there any changes you might recommend to our 504 or Diabetes Care Plans?

- Do you see anything in our child's school schedule that would call for a change of dosing, such as an early or late lunch, gym, or other activity?

"We are incredibly hard on ourselves about any mistake with diabetes. That's easy to do; this condition is unique in that there are many ways to measure our so-called failure."

CHAPTER 5

Reframe Your Diabetes Parent Brain

Benny was diagnosed with T1D one month before he turned two. Like many families with type 1 children, we didn't know of anyone with T1D in our family histories. Our pediatrician sent us to the hospital and life was never the same.

If you're reading this book, you know that "life was never the same" isn't just an expression when a child is diagnosed with T1D. There is a distinct before and after. I truly believe the way we entered the "after" made an enormous difference in our outlook. We were so lucky to have very positive and encouraging experiences right at the start. In fact, my framing of life with T1D started even before Benny's diagnosis.

My career is in media; I'd been a TV health reporter and then a radio show host. Local media people are often asked to MC events and make public appearances. I'm sure you've seen your local anchors at ribbon cuttings and charity events. For many years, before diabetes was in our lives, I acted as the MC of the local JDRF golf tournament! That's where I met families with happy kids who talked about making diabetes part of their everyday life and why it was important to not shelter the kids or hold them back. I interviewed the kids for my radio show and one little boy talked about eating Pop-Tarts! ("Not every day," his mom added as she rolled her eyes.)

When Benny was in the hospital, I reached out to those families. We had a positive and thriving community embrace us immediately.

There were lots of other lucky and positive interactions that first month. A nurse with type 1 stopped by to say hi while Benny was still in the hospital. She spent some time with us and assured me that everything would be OK. My radio listeners were sympathetic and supportive, but quite a few with type 1 were amazing. They were firefighters, bankers, and athletes. They told me to fight my instincts to shelter Benny, and all of them said the best thing that happened to them was their parents letting them pursue big goals and telling them to go for it.

Over the years, we adopted a positive but realistic attitude. There are many people who say, "Diabetes can never stop you!" but we found that it can. A low blood sugar can take you out of a game. A high blood sugar can stop you from feeling well enough to take a test. Technology failures can add time to your day and so can all the mental energy that goes into diabetes. Big picture, of course, diabetes shouldn't stop you from doing what you love. We've tried to be honest but very optimistic with Benny. Diabetes might momentarily stop you, but it's how you move on from there that counts.

I think we've always approached diabetes realistically but with a huge dose of optimism. Because of that, I'm always surprised by the amount of negativity I find these days on much of social media. It's not even about diabetes; it's self-criticism. It's moms like us who want the best for our kids but who are dealing with incredible pressure to be perfect.

Any time you jump into diabetes social media, it won't take long to find a post including the words "mom fail." We are incredibly hard on ourselves about any mistake or mishap with diabetes. That's pretty easy to do; this condition is unique in that there are many ways to measure our so-called failure.

You've got the CGM numbers every five minutes, fingersticks, A1Cs, Time in Range, and any other autoimmune condition you might deal with. Then you've got your child's mental health, development, confidence, and independence to think about. Plus, you're supposed to be taking care of yourself!

Here are some phrases from posts I found in diabetes mom Facebook groups in under ten minutes:

I'm not doing enough. It's all my fault. I'm failing her. My mistake ruined everything. What kind of mother . . . ? I must be the only one who . . . . They're doing it better. How could I forget to . . . ?

Sound familiar? I know I've written at least a few posts over the years that start out with some of those phrases. What's very interesting is that the responses are usually full of support and "been there!" type comments. Think about that for a moment. We're very quick to judge ourselves harshly, but also very quick to support and lift someone else up.

I'd like you to think about how to talk to yourself about your diabetes parenting differently. Doing so in a way more like how you'd support a friend or write a friendly comment on social media.

A helpful way to do this is to reframe how you perceive a situation. Think about the stories we tell ourselves. I have an exercise I'd like you to try that helps me get a little distance from my so-called mistakes and helps me talk to myself in a friendlier way. I call it "reframing my diabetes parent brain."

Think about what happened as a headline. Yes, that's my background as a news reporter coming in, but you can easily do this! What's the headline or summary you'd boil a situation down to if you only had one or two sentences? If you can reframe that into something positive—or at least something where you realize you're not a failure—it may help you take a step in changing your mindset.

Here's an example of a mistake I shared in the first book. Many years ago, we didn't realize that a tubed pump infusion set can fill with sand if you don't cap it. Like many of you, we always threw away the little plastic pitchfork-looking things that come in every box of sets.

I've since interviewed the people who make the infusion sets. The company is called Convatec. They confirm you don't need to cap the sets for much else; the clips are there to keep large debris like sand out. Germs and water can't get through the connection site. It's like the top of an insulin vial. You need the connector needle to poke through.

We discovered what a big problem "large debris" like sand can be after going straight to dinner from the beach. It was the kind of super-casual restaurant where you just throw a coverup over your bathing suit. We ordered and then took out all the diabetes stuff to dose.

Benny tried to reconnect his pump and realized he couldn't. The tubing end just wouldn't go back into the infusion set because it was full of sand!

After trying to flush the site by pouring a bottle of water into it—yes, at the restaurant—we switched out the infusion set. It was stressful and messy and I'm sure the people at the restaurant thought we were bananas.

When I tell this story now, it's easy to see it as a learning experience. We learned that when you remove a tubed pump at the beach, you should cap the infusion set that's still on the body. But at the time, it was upsetting. I felt like I ruined our vacation dinner. Did I? Let's go through the reframing process:

Here's the headline about how I felt at first: "#MomFail! Parents do not properly research or prepare for beach trip. Dinner is delayed. Vacation is ruined."

Here's how I'd reframe it now: "Parents troubleshoot unexpected setback. Happy kids eat dinner. Beach trip is a fun vacation."

We didn't have any of the infusion set clips with us, so my husband, Slade, came up with a great idea. Since the clip is basically the same thing that's at the end of the pump tubing, why not just use that? We change the tubing every three days and

I'd brought extras. He cut off the tubing from the old infusion set we'd just changed, leaving a few inches dangling from the end. He tied a knot and ta-da! New pump clip. I've since shared that trick with dozens of people.

Now I can even add a bonus headline to this one: "MacGyvered solution becomes a big help to other families unfamiliar with an infusion set pitchfork thingee."

In my first book, I related another story where we'd gone to a splash pad on a scorching summer day. It was 100°F and after that fun cooling off, we spent the afternoon inside at home, trying to beat the heat. We didn't yet use a CGM and the afternoon blood sugar check was a shocker: 500 BG! At the time, we were using the Animas Ping pump, which had a remote meter. I bolused Benny from across the room and we checked an hour later. HIGH GLUCOSE! No ketones, thankfully, but something was very wrong. The meter remote was across the room, so I asked Benny to take his pump out of the pouch he wears around his waist. That's when the problem became very clear. He had no pump to take out. Uh-oh!

We had taken the pump off while on the splash pad. I did that a lot around water. The Ping was waterproof, but at that age, Benny always went low anytime swimming or even splashing was involved. Of course, I planned to put the pump back on immediately after. Instead, I'd thrown it in my purse and forgotten about it. All that time I was giving Benny insulin using the remote meter, I'd really been bolusing my purse!

Not a difficult fix—we just needed to get insulin into the kid. We clicked the pump tubing back into the infusion set, did a giant bolus, checked ketones (nope), and refilled Benny's water. That was over ten years ago, and that purse still smells a little like insulin. Gross!

So that's the story. Here's the #MomFail headline: "Mom gets distracted and doesn't pay enough attention. Kid feels lousy because of high blood sugar."

That's technically what happened, but it's just one way of looking at it. I think there's a better way to reframe: "Mom is human and pays attention to more than diabetes. Family has a morning of summer fun and spends the afternoon drinking water and hanging out in the air conditioning."

Same story, different perspective. Let's do one more.

Just before Benny turned seventeen, I turned off all my Dexcom alarms except the urgent low. I'll tell you more about that decision and the process that led us there a little later. Of course, I still check every morning when I wake up! This was a weekend when Benny had the rare chance to sleep late and didn't have to be at work until 2:00 p.m. I woke up at 7:00 a.m., made some coffee, sat down, and looked at the Dexcom.

After cruising steadily around 110 all night (thank you, Control-IQ!), around 6:00 a.m. Benny started going way up. I assumed he'd run out of insulin and was sleeping through the beeping pump. He's a responsible kid, but like most teens, he lets the pump run dry or every once in a while, he forgets to charge it.

I decided to be a great mom and help him out. I planned to grab his pump and refill it, then stealthily put it back on so he can continue to sleep late. He's a pretty heavy sleeper and over the years, I've done my share of ninja moves in the dark. But when I walked in, he was already awake. His pump was full of insulin but out of juice; he'd forgotten to charge it. By the time I walked in, he'd already plugged it in. And he'd also already decided on and delivered a dose to make up for what he'd missed.

I can also add that Benny even got that correction dose right; he came down slowly and evenly and back into range. It's easy to rage bolus (i.e., keep giving insulin because you just want to see the number come down) and crash after a high like that, but he got it right. He even apologized to me for being grumpy!

What's the headline? "Mom doesn't check on pump power before bed—lets teen down by not supporting him? Teen shirks duty—lets pump die?" or "Teen gets diabetes wrong even after living with it for fifteen years?"

I think it's: "Teen is human and forgets to charge pump. Responsibly troubleshoots on his own." Or even "Mom gives teen enough independence to make safe mistakes and learn to troubleshoot."

Take a second and think about your own example. What went wrong recently? What was the story you told yourself? How can you reframe it? It might feel silly, but give it a try!

To be clear, reframing scenarios isn't a magic formula to turn you into a Pollyanna who acknowledges nothing difficult. But reframing has helped me a lot. Years ago, I thought at some point I wouldn't have these feelings of inadequacy; something would "click" and I'd be confident I wasn't doing everything wrong. But with parenting, there is no finish line where someone hands you a medal and says, "Well done!"

I have sixteen years of diabetes parenting under my belt as you're reading this. My son is happy, healthy, and independent. His blood sugar numbers are in a healthy range and our endo approves. All the studies show he should be just fine and live a long healthy life (knock on wood). But I still worry and wonder. Should I have done more? Should I have insisted on tighter control in exchange for less independence?

Why do we still forget things, miss doses, and mess up? We must remember that we're human. I also like what my mother says, "You can't lose. You win or you learn."

I'd also add that as an older mom now—or at least as a mom to older kids (always reframing!)—I can say that I remember a lot less about the exact blood glucose or diabetes care moment-to-moment than I do about the memories of those times. And I guarantee my kids do too. The day we forgot to reconnect the insulin pump, what we really remember is going to the bookstore, the splash pad, and out to lunch. I remember Benny couldn't wait to read his new Elephant and Piggy book while we ate and Lea deciding which book to read out of the three I'd let her buy (instead of the twenty she'd picked out).

If you are unsure or feeling confused, it's important to remember your health care team can be an immense help. Our endocrinologist has been a steady and reassuring presence all these years. He's honest and upfront and points to studies and science. Social media and the diabetes community are terrific for support, but I worry about the amount of medical advice I see from people who got their "degree" on Facebook.

If you listen to my podcast, I always end by saying "be kind to yourself." There's a reason for that. We are our harshest critics. I hope reframing situations or just talking to yourself more like a friend than a critic helps you see how well you're doing. Maybe not perfect, but always learning. And never a #MomFail.

ASK YOUR DOCTOR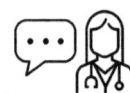

- Are there resources specifically for parents of children with diabetes in our area?

- (Talk about the last #MomFail you had.) Is this a common mistake? Do you have any advice going forward?

- I'm having an issue with . . . and I noticed on social media that some advocate . . . . What are your thoughts on this matter?

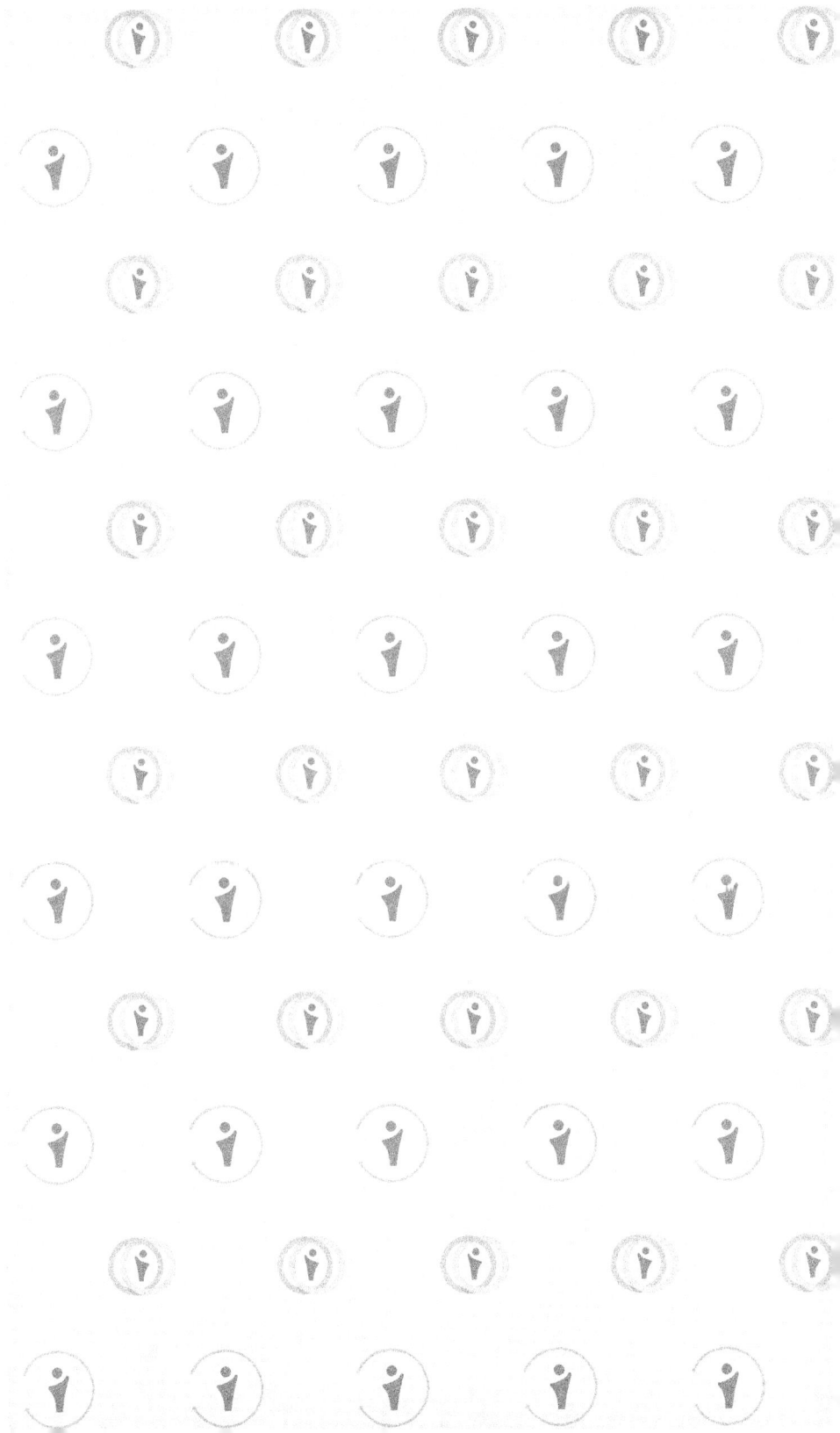

" It's hard to explain to someone without a child with diabetes why pizza is so difficult or why you've invested in a headlamp for overnight checks. Diabetes is an isolating condition. We do much of our toughest work in the middle of the night, alone. "

CHAPTER 6

Making Diabetes Connections

Years ago, a JDRF chapter in St. Louis reached out and asked me to speak. I was still blogging then, and hadn't yet started the podcast, let alone thought about writing a book.

"What do you want me to talk about?" I asked them.

They replied, "What are you most passionate about? What's helped you the most in your family's experience with diabetes?"

That's the story behind the presentation and later the podcast entitled *Diabetes Connections*. I am passionate about finding and connecting with other families touched by diabetes. For me, that started online with the blogs and community I found just after Benny's diagnosis in 2006. It slowly grew into in-person connections locally, two still growing and thriving Facebook groups, the podcast, writing a book, and then another—the book you're reading right now.

Almost everyone wants to make more connections, but there are many who find it very intimidating or don't know where to start. I want to share some ideas and information from that very first presentation and some that I've learned in the years since.

The presentation is called "Diabetes Connections: Why We Need Them, How to Make Them." Let's start with the first part. Why do we need these connections?

Connections are just part of human nature. How many times have you told someone where you're from and their first reaction is to talk about their relative who lives near that area or how they know exactly where that is because their daughter went to college in the next town over? We automatically look for connections and commonalities. It's a basic human need.

It's why, when someone finds out your child has diabetes, they often try to connect in perhaps not the best of ways. I'm sure you've heard, "Oh, my cat has diabetes!" Or "My great-uncle had the bad kind of diabetes, and he didn't take care of himself." Or "I know all about diabetes. Have you heard about the okra and cinnamon cure?"

I believe underneath these not-very-helpful comments are people looking to connect. They want to empathize and show you that you're not alone. Well-meaning, but not particularly helpful. The best diabetes connections are the ones we make with people who understand, who live it, and who can provide resources for each other.

It's hard to explain to someone without a child with diabetes why pizza is so difficult or why you've invested in a headlamp for overnight checks. Diabetes is an isolating condition. We do much of our toughest work in the middle of the night, alone.

Type 1 diabetes is also unique among medical conditions in that the person or caregiver is expected to manage almost every aspect of it on their own. This was brought home to me in an image by Manuel Hernández, formerly of the Diabetes Hands Foundation. It's been estimated that people with diabetes spend about 0.1 percent of their time with a diabetes professional. That decimal point is in the right place! The rest of the time, we're on our own. It's estimated that adds up to nine thousand hours every year of managing diabetes. In a presentation, Hernández showed a big blue circle to indicate the time we spent on our own, with a tiny white line to show the time spent with professional care.[2]

I thought about this image a lot, especially when I felt very alone. Maybe it was during the middle of the night as I hovered over Benny's bed in the dark, fumbling with a flashlight and a meter and trying to figure out why he was 287 or 67. I needed people around me who understood those moments.

Until Benny went to kindergarten, we limited our in-person connections to just JDRF events, which proved valuable, and not just for the good feeling we got every time we went. I remember going to a JDRF-sponsored meetup at a Charlotte Checkers hockey game just a few weeks after Benny's diagnosis. We met a family

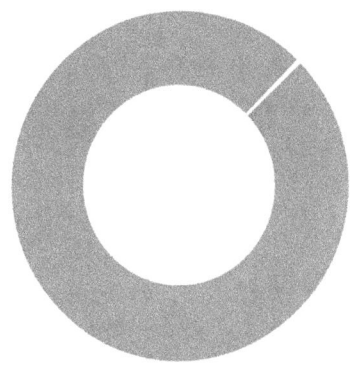

Courtesy of Manuel Hernández

with a child who was a little older than Benny, maybe three years old, and he was wearing a tubed insulin pump like the kind we were considering. He showed us what it looked like and how it connected. It was so helpful! I remember years later going to that same event and showing other families Benny's CGM. That was a full-circle moment.

During that time, I didn't have solid connections in my neck of the woods. Charlotte is a big place and it seemed like all the families we'd met and talked with were in the south part of town, at least forty minutes away from us. But at the tail end of first grade, that changed. Another little boy Benny's age was diagnosed with type 1. And when we came back to school in the fall, I heard there were two more students with type 1.

I wanted to meet the parents, but unlike the boy, who Benny already knew, I had no idea who these families were. Not to be deterred, I gave the school nurse my contact information and asked her to pass it along. I told her I wanted to invite the other moms out to dinner. They responded right away, and we went out together. It was amazing!

Excited about my new connections, I took a photo and put it on Facebook. Almost immediately, I started hearing from my friends who had other friends touched by type 1. I started a "T1D Moms" email list and started setting up dinners once every couple of months. That list grew quickly as word spread. I learned that people are looking to connect but are often waiting for someone else to reach out.

When the email list got big enough to be unwieldy, I started my Charlotte T1D Parents Facebook Group, which now has over one thousand members. It's been a wonderful place to learn, complain, and lift each other up. But the main purpose has been to meet up, to get off the computer and find each other.

If you don't have a local Facebook group, there are a bunch of other ways to find families nearby. Start with JDRF or other diabetes events. Exchange contact information at walks and conferences. It's hard, but try not to be shy! I promise, others are just as hungry for connection as you are. You might be able to plan a coffee meetup right away, or just find out about more opportunities to connect online. Since COVID, many groups have monthly Zoom meetups or chats.

Diabetes camp is another fabulous place to make connections. Your children will probably come home with a list of friends they want to text or otherwise keep in touch with, but you can find other parents there as well. Reach out to your camp staff to see if they have suggestions; sometimes they will hold a parent meeting before or after camp. If you want to organize a meetup after drop-off, something I did for many years, they may help you spread the word.

Camp drop-off meetups are some of my favorites! It's such a marvelous chance for veteran diabetes families to reassure newer ones that everything will be OK. We have a weeklong sleepaway camp in our area and a weekend day camp program. The day camp takes children as young as four years old, so there are some very nervous parents!

Looking for more ideas about connection? I asked my listeners. Here are some of their responses:

We have a parent group that meets once a month. It began at our local teaching hospital through their psychology department. We secured a venue and began meeting last year. We mainly communicate by email and also have a Facebook group.—Clayton

My favorite group is one specifically for type 1 diabetics I found on meetup.com where we get together at different restaurants around the city once a month.—Jodi

I actually found a family that lives about an hour away on a Facebook T1 parent page. We got together for the first time at the zoo a few weeks ago. It is awesome and the whole group bonded quickly. We plan to do more get togethers with our kids as well as just adult outings.—Brooke

I heard a familiar beep across the office, so I went in search of the pump. The "familiar beeps" have led me to several people.—Michelle

I love these stories. I would never have thought to try Meetup.com to find diabetes groups, and it's always great to know that hospitals and endos recognize the importance of patient connections.

It's much easier to connect online, of course. Back when blogging was more popular, there seemed to be an entire network of parent and patient advocates to learn from. We used to call it the Diabetes Online Community (DOC). I'm not sure it really exists today as it was, but there are still lots of valuable places to get great information and support. I found the DOC almost immediately after Benny's diagnosis. The blogs and comments made me feel seen and supported.

A few years later, I joined a Twitter chat called Diabetes Social Media Advocacy. It ran for over ten years every Wednesday at 9:00 p.m. ET with the hashtag #DSMA. It's still around and the organizer recently announced she has something new in mind, so stay tuned!

Like many of you, I'm in a bunch of diabetes Facebook groups. You have to be careful about these. Some of them are so huge that any sense of community gets lost, in my opinion.

I also think that the anonymity of these giant groups makes people feel like they can be very judgmental or even hostile. When you might run into someone at the grocery store, as can happen with a local group, people tend to be much nicer. As I've said before, you also need to be very careful about the medical advice people give in these groups. It's almost all well-meaning, but they don't know your child. Please take any advice you get from Facebook (and from this book!) to your medical team before changing dosing or diabetes management.

My online connections have given me tools to explain things to Benny in ways I would never have thought of otherwise. When he was seven, he started going to regular day camp all summer. I wrote about one of the unexpected challenges he faced, not from diabetes, but from a fellow camper! From my blog:

Benny is at a "regular" day camp now; it's our first time trying this sort of thing. We did a basic diabetes education for the staff and set up a schedule for blood sugar checks, eating and giving insulin. The counselors are just supervising—Benny is doing all the work. Remember, he's 7! We're so proud of him (and, fingers crossed, so far so good).

Except yesterday at dinner, he asked me if poking fingers too many times for BG checks could make someone die. That's what another camper apparently told him (thanks, kid). I suggested that maybe the other boy thought Benny was losing a lot of blood when he tested, which could be dangerous. But that a drop or two a couple of times a day was fine.

He looked skeptical. Thankfully, the amazing Joslin Medalists popped into my head.[3]

I had read about them on Kerri Sparling's blog, *Six Until Me*. The Medalist Program and Study at Joslin[4] recognizes and studies people who have been living with diabetes for at least fifty years. It started in 1948 when the team at Joslin wanted to give their patients an incentive. They started with a 25-year medal and, as more and more people began living longer, healthier lives with diabetes, Joslin expanded the program.

They now give a 50-year, a 75-year, and an 80-year medal! It's also a medical study and a bit of a social group too. I've spoken to many of these amazing medalists for the podcast. It's a very interesting group with a lot of knowledge to share.

I told Benny that there are people living with diabetes for 50 years or more and checking their blood sugar didn't make them die, it helped them live longer.

"I bet they've tested a thousand times," he said.

I laughed and got out the calculator. Benny was diagnosed 5.5 years ago (that's about 2000 days). We do BG checks approximately 7 times a day (often more). He was very impressed to see he's poked his fingers more than 14,000 times and lived to tell the tale.

Having the information about the Joslin Medalists helped me explain something important to Benny in a way that made sense to him.

Sometimes you stumble over information, and sometimes you stumble over new connections. Many people call these "diabetes in the wild." One of my favorites came at a family friend's bat mitzvah. Along with the religious ceremony marking a thirteen-year-old becoming a responsible part of the Jewish community, there is often a big celebration. This was to be a nighttime party with food, dancing, the works. Our diabetes plan for an evening like this is very permissible as long as we know what's going on.

From my blog in 2013:

> I walked Benny over to the kids' table, which was covered in little boxes of candy. We agreed he could have two. We checked out the kids' buffet and decided how many carbs were probably in the pizza and chicken fingers. Math done; it was time to have some fun. Benny likes to hit the dance floor and stay there for as long as he can. He can go a bit high with all the party food, but dancing can make him low. As always, it's a difficult balance.
>
> An hour or so later Benny wasn't feeling well. A quick check showed BG was 400. What happened? We went through what he ate and bolused for. Turns out, he'd had a Sprite. Aha! That was a rare treat we'd agreed to, but he'd forgotten to let us know or to bolus himself. There's a lot going on at these parties, especially for an eight-year-old, so I wasn't too surprised about a rogue soda.
>
> We corrected, but he wasn't bouncing back easily, and I could tell he was sad to miss out on some fun. I looked up and spotted our host's brother, Andrew, across the room. He has type 1! My friend had talked about him before, and I'd met him earlier that day but had completely forgotten until that moment. I told Benny, "See that guy over there? Go show him your pump." Benny looked at me funny for a second, but then he seemed to understand and ran right over.
>
> What a great reaction! Andrew, who is also a pediatrician, took his pump out of his pocket and high-fived Benny. They even had the same Animas pump.

I could see them talking excitedly to each other, then they ran upstairs to the party photo booth and took ridiculous pictures with wild hats, sunglasses, and fake mohawks.

Thank you, Dr. Andrew Lubell, from the bottom of my heart. It's hard to express how much something like this means to me and my family. You took my son from being sad at a celebration, to being happy and right back to having fun. You gave him something joyful to consider about diabetes.

And you rock that neon mohawk.[5]

There's no way to plan for an amazing "in the wild" encounter like that one. But it's an example of why seeking out a connection is so important.

I know I make it sound easy; let's acknowledge that it's not. Setting up dinners and meetings takes work. Not everyone is as comfortable as I am with reaching out. But my local group is one of the best things I've ever been part of. Those connections have helped me manage our lives with diabetes since the day Benny was diagnosed. It really is worth your time and effort.

A local group is an incredible source of information and support you can't get anywhere else. We can talk about everything diabetes, like giving shots in public, handling situations at school and local restaurants, vacations, traveling, and all the regular stuff.

In real life, we can assist each other. We can recommend babysitters, local camp programs we know will accommodate our kids, be a backup plan for nervous grandparents who are watching the kids, and much more. We live in a community where there are very few people who've been here for generations. Charlotte is a town with a lot of transplants. If you don't have family nearby, your diabetes mom friends are happy to help fill in the gaps.

As parents, we're always trying to help our children connect, but we can forget how much we need the same support. Our children are amazing, but their diabetes perspectives are not ours. Benny needs his own peers just as much as I do, whether it's from diabetes camps, JDRF conferences, or a pen pal. As a parent of a child with type 1, I also need to know I'm not alone. Simply going to lunch or dinner, having coffee together, being with people who just get it, helps in a way little else can.

I surveyed my podcast listeners a few years back. They were almost all looking for diabetes connections, but most didn't know where to find them in real life. It's one reason I started a project you'll be hearing more about very soon. I'm calling it Club 1921, a place to find and list diabetes events. It features everything from mom meetups to big conferences, online workshops, and professional education sessions. Stay tuned for more on Club 1921, named, of course, after the year insulin was discovered.[6]

Get in touch. Stay in touch. The connections you make now and sustain won't make your child's and your family's experience with diabetes easy, stress free, or a walk in the park. But it will make it so much better. We are not alone. We need each other. To learn, to laugh, to cry, to embarrass our children in silly ways, and to share when they make us so proud. You get it. So do I. Let's connect and find out how strong we all are together.

ASK YOUR DOCTOR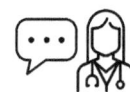

- Are there any local groups for parents of children with diabetes?

- Does your staff ever have meetups or educational programs for families?

- What are some ways other local parents connect with the diabetes community?

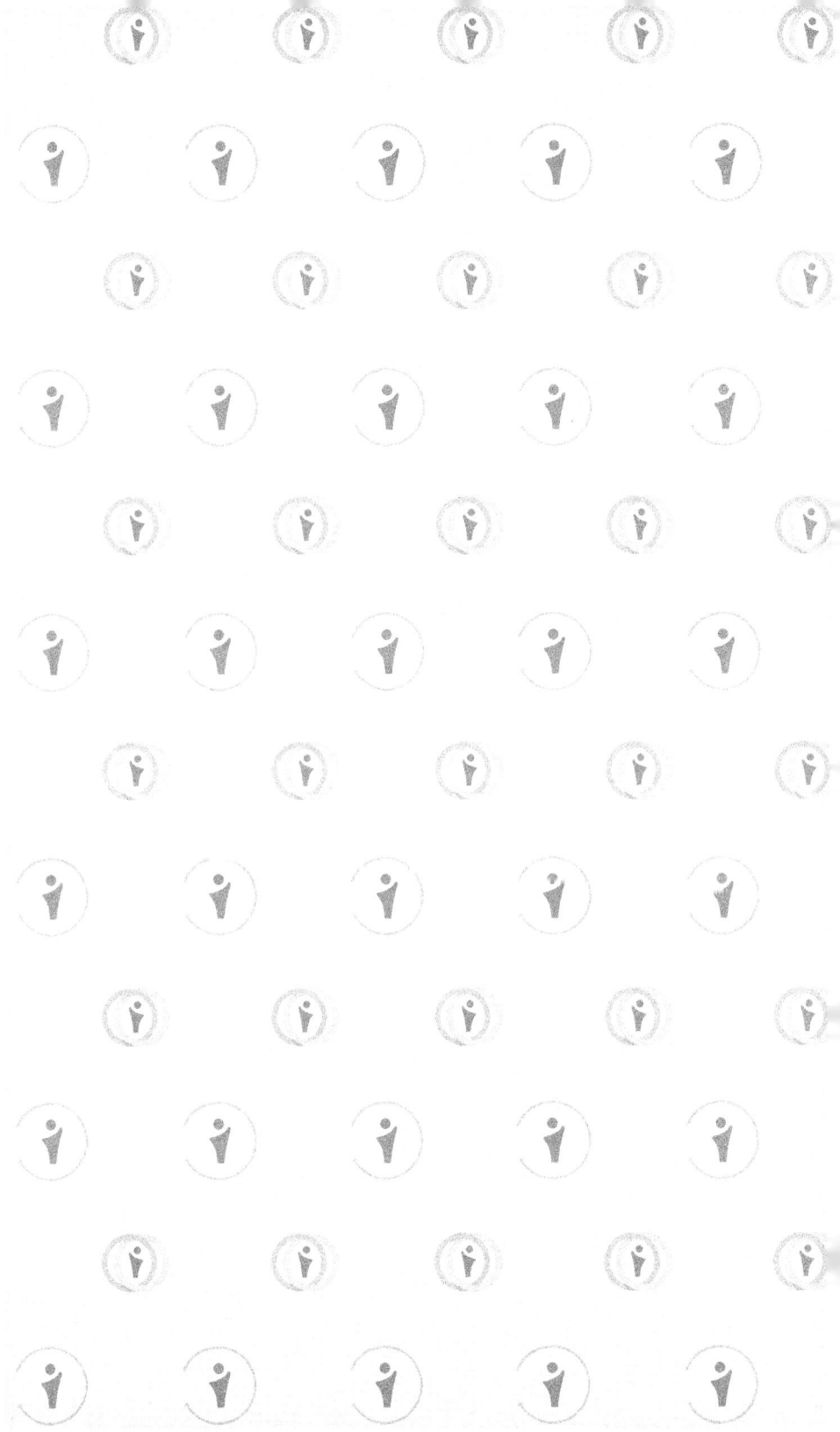

❝ 'Technology and tools are useful and powerful when they are your servant and not your master,' stated educator & author Stephen Covey. A CGM is a tool, and it's up to us to figure out how to use it in a way that improves our experience with diabetes and helps our children thrive. **❞**

CHAPTER 7

Our CGM Timeline

I t's hard to overstate how continuous glucose monitoring has changed the game in the last ten years.

We know the difference firsthand because we went the first seven years of diabetes with no CGM. From ages two to nine, we relied on fingersticks for that part of Benny's management. That meant seven to ten pokes on a regular day—more if he wasn't feeling well. We did one glucose check overnight (again, more if Benny was sick or something was wonky) and felt satisfied we had enough information.

Once we put the CGM on, we realized we'd missed a billion highs and lows. We now had a tool that could help us more accurately and dynamically manage diabetes. Information makes an enormous difference with a condition like T1D; we now had a way to get a 24-7 panorama when we'd previously been limited to snapshots.

There's a quote credited to Stephen Covey, author of *The 7 Habits of Highly Effective People,*[7] that really speaks to me about how we use CGM. "Technology and tools are useful and powerful when they are your servant and not your master," he said. A CGM is a tool, and it's up to us to figure out how to use it in a way that improves our experience with diabetes and helps our children thrive.

Before we dig into everything, I want to let you know Dexcom is a long-time sponsor of my podcast. They don't tell me what to say and no one from the company has seen this chapter (or any of this book) before publication. Even so, I think it's important to disclose these relationships.

We absolutely love using a CGM and it's hard to imagine going without it these days. The biggest value for us was not so much peace of mind; we weren't terrified of diabetes while using fingersticks. It was more about gaining access to all that valuable information. These days, CGM helps make possible AID pump systems, which are truly life changing. Using one for the past two and a half years has allowed Benny to think about diabetes less while getting more Time in Range.

Let's take a minute and talk about CGM, especially about why it's different from fingersticks. A fingerstick is measuring the glucose in your blood. A CGM measures glucose in the fluid just under the skin, called interstitial fluid. These are both accurate ways to measure, but they won't always match. Glucose moves from the blood vessels and capillaries first and then to interstitial fluid. Usually, the CGM number lags just behind a fingerstick. You can also expect to see a bigger difference between the two when glucose is changing rapidly, such as after eating or taking insulin.

CGM is a great tool, but I worry about the fear and anxiety I've seen sprout up around it in the last few years. Before I say more about that, I think it will be helpful to share some of our stories and mistakes around continuous glucose monitoring.

Please note: I'm focusing almost exclusively on Dexcom, because that's what we've used. However, the Medtronic and Abbott FreeStyle Libre CGMs have many of the same features. Eversense is another brand of CGM available in the US, but at the time of publishing this book, it is not yet approved for children. Share is a brand name for Dexcom. In this book, I'm using it interchangeably with (lowercase) share to mean sending numbers from a user's CGM to a caregiver's phone or interface, regardless of brand or software system.

We started with the Dexcom G4 PLATINUM in December 2013. It wasn't yet approved for anyone under eighteen, but our doctor wrote us an off-label prescription. A few months later, the G4 PLATINUM pediatric version was approved. The only difference was you had to scroll through a couple of warning screens on the receiver.

You may know that Dexcom launched in 2006, and Medtronic had a sensor out even before that. Why didn't we start sooner?

The accuracy really wasn't what it is today and the first sensors only lasted three days. Even the G4 was only approved for seven days of use. Benny had used a pump since age two, and I was reluctant to put something else on his body until I could be sure it would be worth it. There was also the question of what he wanted; he was old enough to start having a say in these types of decisions.

I also had an embarrassing misunderstanding of how CGMs worked. The turning point for me, and for Benny, came as it so often does, after we met someone in the diabetes community who was using the technology.

For me, that someone was Tom Brobson. In 2013, Brobson was JDRF's National Director of Research Investment Opportunities. He was traveling the country talking to people about something JDRF was doing called the "Artificial Pancreas Project." Of course, this was the framework for funding and research that would lead to everything from Medtronic's 670G to the Tandem Control IQ system Benny's used since 2020 and to Omnipod 5, just approved this year.

Back in 2013, I wrote:

> I try not to get too excited about diabetes "breakthroughs" or technology announcements. Years ago, before I even had a personal connection to type 1, I covered the Glucowatch and Exubera inhaled insulin as a TV health reporter. Never heard of them? Yeah, they didn't work out so well.
>
> When Benny was diagnosed in 2006, I was a bit skeptical of the new technology our doctor talked about.

Called the artificial pancreas, he described it as an insulin pump, a continuous glucose monitor (CGM) and a computer. They'd work together to control blood sugar automatically, just like a working pancreas. It sounded great, but I was wary of getting my hopes up. Six and a half years later, I think I'm ready to let them start to fly.

Of course, it would be another six and a half years until Benny would use one of these systems! But something else Tom shared that day made a more immediate impact:

I'm embarrassed to admit this after years of being in the diabetes world, but I always thought a CGM had some sort of tubing. Newsflash: it does not. This became clear in my questions to Tom and he was pretty surprised at my misunderstanding. He ripped off his shirt (OK, he rolled up his sleeve) to show me the CGM. There's no tubing and it sits almost flat on the skin.[8]

OK, go ahead and laugh. What did I think tubing would be for? In the days before social media, it was hard to see photos of diabetes tech. We went to almost every local JDRF event back then and I remember seeing pumps and, of course, lots of meters. I can't recall ever seeing a CGM.

Tom was happy to show me his sensor and told me that knowledge from the CGM more than made up for having another "thing" on his body (he also wore a pump). After noting my confusion, he didn't mind showing me what the CGM was all about, and I'm so grateful. I'm also grateful he didn't mind me telling the version of the story where he rips his shirt off.

I told Benny about meeting Tom and showed him a video I took, but he wasn't super interested. He was doing just fine, so my husband and I agreed to let it go for a while. I met Tom in April 2013 and at an endo visit that fall, Benny brought up a CGM totally unprompted. He'd seen them at diabetes camp and wanted to know more. And just like that, we got a prescription and had it in our hands in a few weeks.

You may recall from the first book that we started Benny's insulin pump the week of July fourth, when we were away at my parents' house. We don't live close, but I felt the family support would more than make up for the distance from home. It would have worked out just fine, except that we forgot to pack a crucial part of the pump refill process. It's a long (and already told) story. Suffice it to say, after a family-wide freakout, we found what we needed and carried on.

If you remember that, it may not surprise you that we started the Dexcom over the winter break on another visit to the grandparents. I wanted to start CGM while Benny was out of school, just to make sure we all got used to it. Remember, this was before Share, so it was just about learning to insert the sensor and use the receiver that Benny would take with him.

Here's what I wrote in January 2014:

First impressions? We love it. A CGM gives copious amounts of data, which is incredibly useful to a person with diabetes. It also alarms when BG is going too high or too low.

I'm impressed with how well it stays on. No issues at all with it coming off so far. We started while visiting my parents in Florida and Benny spent a lot of time in the pool. That was a problem with insets in the past, so I was prepared for it to come off ("just make sure you dive for the transmitter!!"). Even with 4 days of swimming for several hours at a time, it stuck fast. We use Skin-Tac as a prep but, so far, no tape over the sensor transmitter.

I am disappointed that I can't use the receiver on my nightstand or anywhere in my room. It's just too far away and even near my door is out of range. When we realized that, we hoped Benny would keep it with him while he slept, but we spooked him the first night out. We set the high threshold too low the first night (before the CGM was really calibrated) and it alarmed three times, waking him up and freaking him out, before I just turned it off.

(My cousin is reading this and laughing. Her son with type 1 recently started on the same CGM. She left me a voice mail that I didn't listen to that first night. What did it say? "Set the alarms higher than usual. It will alarm more than you want, before it's calibrated.")

I'm also disappointed with how big and scary the inserter is. So far, Slade has put the sensor on Benny. I'm going to call my educator and see if she can spare an inserter for me to practice with. This part is harder than we thought it would be. After six and a half years on a pump, I guess I thought he'd be used to all the stabbing insertions. We don't use numbing cream for the inset any longer and, when he needs to, he does them himself. But the CGM needle is larger and seems to hurt a bit more.

The second insertion was pretty stressful—Benny almost decided he didn't want a CGM anymore. But he toughed it out. The third change went better; he really likes having it and this was his call all the way. I've been asking him to think about a CGM for two years. I thought he was set this summer, but at our August checkup, he said no. I didn't bring it up again, but in November, he told Dr. V he was ready. I'm glad I didn't push. I can't imagine how tough the sensor changes would be if he wasn't on board.[9]

The G4 didn't use Bluetooth. It worked via radio frequency (RF), so it wasn't too difficult to find a spot outside Benny's bedroom that would pick up the signal. We've found RF to be a bit less fussy than Bluetooth. We moved the receiver into the hallway for the night and left it there for the next couple of years. This helped keep alarms from waking him up, and it was close enough to my room so that I could hear it.

Even when Benny moved to a phone, it was placed in the hallway overnight. We had a no-cell-phone-in-your-bedroom-at-night rule for both kids. Having said that, it can be difficult for Bluetooth to connect through a closed door or too far away. If you can't connect, there are lots of ways to limit phone use to just the apps you need overnight. I think it's too tempting for kids to have their phones nearby while they sleep. I can barely put mine down sometimes!

We agreed that when Benny went back to school, he'd use the CGM in place of fingersticks. We always scheduled BG checks around the class schedule and saw no reason for that to change. Going forward, instead of doing a fingerstick, at the appointed time, he'd simply look at the receiver. He was in fourth grade and was still showing his teacher his BG number a couple of times a day.

We never had Benny go to the nurse for care. Starting in kindergarten, his teachers or other helpers would oversee his diabetes management. Part of that was because we didn't have a full-time school nurse (not uncommon where we live) and also because Benny had already had diabetes for four years when he started kindergarten. With strict supervision, he could use his insulin pump and check his blood sugar. The Dexcom would just be a new tool to work into this successful routine. It worked well—for about two weeks. That's when Benny lost the receiver.

From my blog in January 2014:

I am so excited to report all about our first two weeks using the Dexcom CGM. But first I have to tell you about how we almost lost it. Yes, already.

A continuous glucose monitor (CGM) has three parts. The transmitter and sensor connect to each other and are attached to your body. The receiver is separate and can be carried in your pocket or put in a case and worn on a belt. It's about the size of an iPod touch.

Tuesday, our school had a two-hour delay because of the cold weather. Even with the extra time, it was still chaos in my house when Benny left for the bus stop. That's when I realized I hadn't taken one last peek at the Dexcom. Did he have it on?

I didn't see the receiver in the house, but I couldn't shake the feeling, so I texted our wonderful school nurse. She confirmed no CGM receiver, but Benny was sure he left the house with it. So where was it?

At this point, I was at work about 30 minutes from school and home. Slade walked to the bus stop and back. He looked in a few obvious places at home (under the bed, in the hamper, by the computer) but held off the urge to turn the place upside down.

Finally, after an hour that seemed like a week, transportation staff found the receiver on the bus. The angels sang and no calls were made that day to insurance companies or diabetes supply groups! Slade drove down to Charlotte to pick up what we assumed would be a case with a broken snap.

Nope, turns out the snaps are fine, the case is fine. How did it come off? No idea. Of course, now we're double-checking the snap when Benny leaves the house (he's thrilled) and I'm looking into a backup case or two.

Who's coming up with the "find my CGM" app? We'll be the first to sign up![10]

The next big change came in December 2014, with the Share Cradle, which I mentioned in the chapter 3 about sleepovers. The Share Cradle was a decent idea, but not especially useful on the go. We used it at night, plugging the phone in and keeping the cradle in the hallway outside Benny's room.

We got the next version of Share in mid-2015. This meant the receiver could signal Benny's phone and then share to our phone via Wi-Fi. We didn't use it much because I didn't want to get my ten-year-old a phone! Finally, in fifth grade, we got him one, but he rarely used it. It's hard to imagine now, right?

The first time I remember leaning on Share was toward the end of the fifth grade, when Benny's class went on a field trip to Washington, D.C. I wrote about that as "The Big Field Trip" in the first book. Here's a Facebook post I shared at the time, to a diabetes mom group:

> He's off! B left around 6:00 a.m. for D.C. I just got a text from my neighbor's wife (my neighbor is the dad in charge of Benny's group) thanking me for trusting him with Benny's care. She said they're glad they can help. How nice was that?! Also, I don't know how people remote monitor on a regular basis. I am going to have to train myself not to look at the damn phone every five minutes! ☺

Isn't that cute?

By the way, if you can't imagine *not* staring at your phone or smart watch every five minutes, you're not alone. I think that's very common for anyone who starts Dexcom and Share at the same time. Most people are able to stop looking so frequently as the novelty wears off. If you're struggling with that, I have some ideas to help in the next chapter.

Through middle school, we gradually used Share and Follow more and more. We still didn't use it for the four weeks of summer camp—no Wi-Fi there and he'd been going since 2011, before he'd even had Dexcom. While Share was helpful, we didn't feel nervous without it.

One of the best parts of Share/Follow was that it helped us troubleshoot using a lot more data. If Benny called from a sleepover with dosing questions, we could look at a much bigger picture to help figure out how much insulin he might give for dinner or how much of a correction to give (or withhold) before bed. It also helped us to jump on highs and lows much earlier than before.

Since the spring of 2018, we've used the Dexcom G6. This was a terrific step forward for Benny's independence. I mentioned the huge inserter for previous versions; this one is much less scary and easier to operate. Benny can easily place the sensor himself. In the over four years since switching, he's done every insertion. The G6 also doesn't need to be calibrated, which meant no nagging my teenager to remember to do a fingerstick every morning and every night.

This book is due to come out around the same time the Dexcom G7 is expected to roll out to consumers. Libre and Medtronic are also stepping up their CGM offerings, and there are over thirty new CGM systems in various stages of development around the world! It's an exciting time for a piece of tech that has literally changed the way we look at diabetes.

ASK YOUR DOCTOR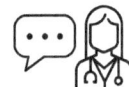

- Tell me about the options for CGM. Which do you think might be best for my child and why?

- Knowing the age and body weight of my child, are there any places you'd recommend we insert the CGM sensor?

- How do your patients who thrive with CGM seem to use it?

“ We don't have to sacrifice communication and empathy for a little bit more Time in Range. ”

CHAPTER 8

Conversations around CGM

A round the same time the G6 came out, I noticed something interesting in my local parent group. No longer waiting weeks or months to start CGM, children were being diagnosed with T1D and sent home from the hospital with a Dexcom. Charlotte, North Carolina, was one of the pilot programs for early CGM adoption in newly diagnosed kids.

How did we find out about the new program? There wasn't an announcement. Instead, we suddenly started seeing basic questions in our group that hadn't come up before. Questions like: "What do the arrows mean?" "Can my child shower with the Dexcom on?" And "Can my child sleep with the Dexcom on?" There was also a lot of panic about troubleshooting Dexcom issues and with not knowing how to perform fingerstick blood glucose checks.

We quickly figured out something had changed. It seemed the Dexcom education was coming on top of the already incredibly info-dense diabetes education. The two together made for some very confusing times. My group was more than happy to help, but I think this issue is creating a lot of stress for newer families, something CGM is supposed to alleviate!

I love CGM. It's an incredible tool, but you must know how to use it. If you're reading this book, you likely remember those confusing first days or weeks after diagnosis. Some say it's like drinking from a fire hose. I say it's like trying to drink from an ocean! There's just so much information. To then have your child wear a CGM and share numbers immediately can go smoothly for some, but it can be very confusing and overwhelming for others.

I've looked at studies around parenting and CGM use and there doesn't seem to be a consensus. Some show an increase in the parent's anxiety, others show it goes down. Another shows more family tension after starting CGM, especially in parents of teens with type 1.

One study in the American Diabetes Association's (ADA) journal, *Diabetes*, caught my eye. "In summary, while not reaching statistical significance, results suggest that caregivers have different reasons for starting CGM in their children which may be found to be related to their emotional state."[11]

In other words, parents of children with type 1 diabetes are individuals with different needs, expectations, and parenting styles. So rather than tell you what I think you should do and how you should share, I'd like to pose some questions that may help you figure out what works best for your family.

Please keep in mind, I'm not debating whether your child should wear a CGM. This is about using remote monitoring to help your child with diabetes management while also strengthening your relationship for the long term. I promise, we don't have to sacrifice communication and empathy for a little bit more Time in Range.

Why do I want to remote monitor?

This sounds like a dumb question, right? Why wouldn't you want to see your child's blood glucose numbers? But I'd like you to think specifically about what might change in your family's diabetes management. Is there a problem you're trying to solve or a particular situation you want to troubleshoot?

It's hard to imagine how different it would have been to have used a CGM with a share capability when Benny was first diagnosed. How would I have answered this question? When he was a toddler, I'd have said to help other caregivers as needed. We were lucky to have an amazing day care and babysitters, but seeing the numbers would have made some of those phone calls a little easier. I think it would also have been helpful to avoid some lows. Toddlers are very unpredictable and can drop fast. It would have been nice to have a warning at 70 before we noticed Benny looked woozy and before we checked to find that he was much lower. Never any emergencies, but we had quite a few lows under 55 before starting CGM.

In elementary school, I would have said we wanted it to help him during sports, after school at friends' homes, and to help us all sleep better. That last one is tricky, though. Some studies show children get more sleep with CGM but parents get less.[12] That makes sense to me; I can only imagine how many highs and lows we slept through before CGM. But waking up to every single slightly out-of-range number isn't healthy either. We talked to our endo to come up with a range that kept Benny safe and allowed me to get some rest. There is nothing wrong with increasing the threshold of a high alarm on a night when the parent is exhausted. Your health matters too. Using an AID system has completely changed our overnights, but how you will balance sleep and diabetes management is still worth thinking about before starting any remote monitoring system.

Who else will get access to my child's numbers?

This is a tricky one and I'd urge you to think through sharing with everyone who cares for your child.

We shared with my mother for a few years. While we were visiting in Florida, we went away for an overnight and she watched the kids. It made sense to add her as a follower to Benny, but we forgot to remove her when we returned home. She lives over 600 miles away. The next time that urgent low blared in the middle of the night, guess who called me? We set some rules (more on that) and she stayed as a follower until a few years later.

What about school staff? This is a very personal decision and I'd be careful about rushing into it. Most teachers and nurses are excellent about this, and I understand that having people in the building knowing your child's glucose numbers all day long may give you more peace of mind. But I have heard many stories about staff that overreacts, pulling kids from class for every alarm or, even worse, being judgmental about highs and lows. I think it would be difficult to take away the follow "power" from a school nurse or helper, so be sure that's something you want to start.

We have never shared with the school, for several reasons. The first year it would have been practical was sixth grade, the first year of middle school. Benny was just starting to get more independent with diabetes management at school and didn't want anyone looking over his shoulder. We agreed it wasn't necessary for him, but reserved the right to revisit. We've never changed our minds.

If you share with anyone, I think it's worth at least a conversation about expectations and communication before you start.

What does my child think about it?

No matter the age, I'm a big fan of talking to our kids about these decisions. Even in middle school, when almost any conversation would cause an automatic eye roll and a "whatever," just knowing that I cared enough to ask made a difference. Benny would almost always tell me what was on his mind, even if it was two days later in the car or just before bed. He knew I would listen.

Of course, this depends on age. For a younger child, I think it's a good idea to explain who can see their numbers and why. We got great advice early on to avoid phrases like, "So we can keep you safe," but say instead, "So you can feel good and play." We didn't want to teach Benny to fear diabetes, especially when he was a toddler!

For elementary school children, I think it's a good idea to have a conversation with them and their health-care team together, if you can. At the very least, decide as a family how you'll share at school and with whom. Then present that plan to the school. That way, your child is on board and knows the expectations.

If your child tells you they don't want to share at school or with other caregivers, encourage them to talk to you about why. Is there one staff member who's a little too overreactive? Or are they embarrassed by beeping or interruptions? There are lots of ways to manage at school that can be a little more low-key. Going back to only looking at Dexcom numbers at certain times of day, raising the high alarm just a little bit (ask your endo), and encouraging staff to let your child lead are a few ways to help shy kids feel more comfortable.

What are your family's "rules of engagement"?

What's the plan for when the CGM alarm goes off? Talking through the possibilities has been a tremendous help for us. As Benny got older, we talked about what range he'd set on the CGM and what range I would set on mine. His range was a bit tighter. After all, he was the one responsible for taking action. My high alarm was set higher and my low was set a bit lower. I love that CGMs give you the options to customize alarms!

Here's what we agreed to for middle school: If Benny was very high, let's say above 300, I'd text him after thirty minutes. In my mind, that's more than enough time to troubleshoot and treat If he was above 200 for more than an hour, I'd do the same. If he was below 80 (but higher than 60) for more than half an hour, same thing. And the same if he was below 60 for fifteen minutes. To us, that seemed reasonable for a child who'd been living with diabetes for ten years and was already relatively independent.

What about his side of things? Our 504 plan indicated he could text me anytime, but middle school is busy and there's a lot going on. I didn't want to overload him, so we agreed that for high BG, as long as I saw the arrow turn in the time I mentioned in the previous paragraph, he didn't have to text back at all.

For the lows, he had fifteen minutes to get back to me—all

he had to do was text "I'm on it," or "Treated." If I didn't get that quick text back within the times we'd agreed to, and I didn't see the numbers change, I'd call the school.

If I still couldn't reach him, I promised I'd drive to school and yell out of the window, "My baby! My baby!" This is a fantastic threat I've used with both children if texts went unanswered, diabetes or not. I'm proud to say I never had to do it. But I promise I would have. Maybe I'll do it just one time before Benny graduates.

For younger or newly diagnosed children, you might decide on different parameters. I would likely have communicated sooner and within a tighter range during elementary school. But too tight a range can cause issues as well.

I had a friend who would check her son's CGM values all day long during school hours and text several times a day if his BG was high. Here's the problem with that: insulin is slow, and it lasts a lot longer in the body than most people think. How long is a school day? If your child is correcting three times a day and bolusing for all the carbs, that can create a low BG situation just when it's time to get on the school bus home. It happened to us quite a few times before we caught on.

Another tough fact about remote monitoring is remembering that a CGM is about fifteen minutes behind the actual blood glucose. It can also be slower to catch up when coming down from highs or going up from lows.

I've shared some of our ranges here and I know by doing so I'm opening myself up to criticism. That's fine. I don't think the exact numbers and ranges are the point. It's about making a plan and following it. I promise you, it wasn't easy to keep from texting Benny for every high and low, especially that first year of middle school! But if I'd done that, I don't think we'd have the open and honest relationship we have today. This system works for me and Benny and I'm confident it's been the right way for us to go about it. After nearly sixteen years of diabetes, I have a happy and healthy kid who's independent but still wants to spend time with me. I have prioritized our relationship over "perfect" blood sugars, and I'm happy with that decision.

In Benny's final year of high school, I have turned off all Dexcom alerts (except urgent low) and he's now 100 percent independent in terms of day-to-day care. It's what we've been working for all this time. It's great. And also, I hate it.

What will I do when technology fails?

We have been very fortunate that Dexcom sensors work well for Benny. In the four plus years we've used the G6, I'd say we get the full ten days at least 90 percent of the time with great accuracy. There was one time when we had a day full of failure and, of course, it was when I was heading out of town.

In October 2019, I was excited about attending the first-ever She Podcasts conference. The morning I was set to leave, Benny had no school and was due for a sensor change. As I was packing up the last of my things, he yelled, "Mom, the sensor failed!" It had conked out during the warmup. He was already getting another sensor ready, so I started loading up my car.

That sensor failed too.

Because the Dexcom reads values every five minutes, we had always been told to wait at least that amount of time between sensor changes to make sure the transmitter knows we're starting a new sensor and not trying to reuse the old one. We waited a good twenty minutes, then tried another sensor. No go.

Amazingly, I had two sensors left. We rarely have this much of a stockpile. I didn't want to risk it; we so rarely have sensor issues I assumed something was wrong with the transmitter. I called Dexcom and they transferred me to Tandem to troubleshoot. The person I spoke with was terrific and thorough and walked us through a bunch of troubleshooting steps. I, however, was getting impatient; I was supposed to be on the road already!

Under her instruction, we put in a fourth sensor, and I got ready to head out. I told Benny to call me and let me know the status and that I would continue the conversation on the road with Tandem if need be. Benny was fourteen at the time and just wanted to be left alone to enjoy his day off from school. My husband would be home later that day, so I got in the car and left for Atlanta.

That fourth sensor failed as well. My husband has type 2 diabetes and occasionally uses the Libre CGM. Benny decided he'd rather wear that than fingerstick, which was fine by me. I spent more time on the phone with Tandem while I drove to my conference. We decided it was likely a transmitter issue and they agreed to send replacements.

Benny wore the Libre for the rest of that week. At the time, it didn't have a remote monitoring function. After we received the new transmitter and sensor replacement, the Dexcom issue was resolved. It was a frustrating experience, especially when I was away from home, but being without Share and Follow for a week didn't change our plans. School, sports, social stuff—Benny did it all. Even if we didn't have the Libre, he would have done fingersticks. Not ideal, but easily doable.

Sometimes the issue is system wide. A few years ago, on New Year's Eve, there was an issue with Dexcom Share. The user's phone or receiver was working fine. However, the Follow app didn't work. It was a complete fiasco. The mainstream media coverage and social media commentary about this matter went on for weeks.

While I think Dexcom could have handled the situation better, especially in terms of communication, it saddened me to see so many parents react with panic and alarm. I'm sure I would have felt the same if we hadn't spent so much time feeling safe and happy without CGM. But servers can fail, sensors will fall off, and companies will sometimes not send enough supplies. To me, it's important to be prepared. Make sure you have a working blood glucose meter and you know how to use it. Talk to your endo about how many times you might check BG with a meter and create a backup plan. That way, if the CGM or just the Share goes down, you'll be better prepared.

What if my child doesn't want to wear it?

I once had an argument with another parent about letting our kids choose their technology. He told me that I wouldn't let my child say no to a cast if they broke their arm or to chemotherapy if they had cancer. So why would I allow them to ever be without a CGM?

I strongly disagree with this way of thinking. Let me say one more time. I *love* CGM. But people with diabetes have very few choices. They must put insulin in their body, and they must measure blood glucose. No choice for those two tasks. But in my opinion, how those tasks are accomplished is up to the person with diabetes. And yes, a child can make those body autonomy decisions.

Of course, age and other factors come into play here. I didn't ask two-year-old Benny if he wanted an insulin pump. But I let eight-year-old Benny decide about his CGM. As a parent, you make the rules in your house and ultimately these decisions are up to you, but I urge you to present all diabetes technology as options and not edicts.

I'm not above rewarding or offering incentives (aka bribes) for trying a CGM. Give it two weeks or a month and here's a LEGO set or a shopping trip. In my experience, a CGM makes so many things easier that most children with diabetes prefer using it over having multiple fingersticks every day. As long as their endo believes they are safe and healthy, forcing any technology can backfire in the long run. And I stand by my opinion that a CGM is not the same as chemotherapy.

How can I stop staring at the numbers?

Once you get Share, it's tough to stop looking at the numbers. We've had it for nearly nine years and I still struggle with this. It's controversial to even mention that this might be a problem; I know people who have their child's BG numbers on display on screens all over their homes. This is all so new that there aren't any studies, but I can't imagine we're going to find out that seeing

BG numbers in our face around the clock is going to make a meaningful difference to diabetes management, and it may even be harmful in some unexpected ways.

If you're just starting out with Share, you may decide to look at it only at certain times of the day. The alarms will let you know when you or your child will need to take action. Once you do, keep in mind that insulin can be slow and that CGM can lag behind, especially to reflect rising BG after lows. That means there's no use checking every five minutes to see if a high is coming down or checking every minute to confirm a low is under control.

You can also move the Follow app to a different screen on your phone. I moved mine off the home page ages ago.

If you are using screens or other tools in very visible places, consider your child's age and stage. It might be great when they're three and you're trying to stay on top of volatile BG while also caring for a child who needs your help with everything! But it may not be as effective for your eleven-year-old who really doesn't want such a visible reminder of diabetes everywhere they look.

Again, I'm not saying you shouldn't use or rely on the CGM information. But there is a difference between using a tool like this to help our children thrive and letting it consume our thoughts to where, if we can't see the numbers for even fifteen minutes, panic sets in. Diabetes technology should make our lives easier, not add another layer of stress.

What's next?

When Benny started with a CGM in 2013, there were about 60,000 people using a Dexcom worldwide, according to the company. In 2022, it's estimated that more than 4.5 million people worldwide are using a Dexcom, Libre, or Medtronic CGM. This technology isn't going anywhere, and use will continue to grow.

It's amazing to me to look back and remember that we routinely did eight to ten fingersticks a day, every day, and more on sick days or when things were wonky. By the time Benny was nine and started on CGM, his fingertips looked horrible. When they got wet, you could really see all the pinpricks; even dry, they were pitted and marked up. It's amazing to me that now his fingertips are smooth and clear. I never imagined that would happen. What a joy!

I'm thrilled with Control-IQ and if we ever figure out the access and affordability issue, AID systems and remote monitoring are going to become standard care. Even so, I still think it's about more than numbers and Time in Range. Taking a few minutes to think this through and communicate with your child will help with more than diabetes management. It will help your relationship and your peace of mind.

ASK YOUR DOCTOR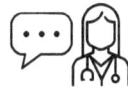

- Are there conversations you suggest we have before we start remote monitoring?

- Do you think it's time to revisit our CGM monitoring routine now that my child is older than when we started?

- What should we know in case the CGM technology fails?

“ You can have highs and lows
with diabetes wherever you are.
Why let that keep you stuck at
home? Go see the world! ”

CHAPTER 9

Vacation Adventures

We love to travel, and diabetes certainly keeps it interesting! We've been lucky enough to have some wonderful vacations and experiences, even with diabetes mistakes and problems.

First, you should know that I am a big vacation planner. That's part of the fun, for me, especially for theme parks. It always pays off; you wait in far fewer lines, you know when you'll eat, and everyone is less grumpy.

When Benny had just turned thirteen, we had a long-planned trip to the Orlando parks over winter break, including two days at Universal. On the first day, we arrived at the park early and had breakfast. Eating breakfast at a theme park is usually a colossal waste of time, but I had a plan. And my family does better with a proper meal on a day like this. Business as usual, we bolused for breakfast and we were ready to go. Just as we were clearing the table, Benny noticed his infusion set was leaking.

I handed him the diabetes bag and he got everything out to change it. He looked up at me, "Mom, where are the insets?"

At this point in our management, Benny wasn't as independent as he is now, almost five years later. At this age, we were both sort of packing the diabetes bag, which is a terrible way to go about things. I thought he was checking and repacking it, and he assumed I was in charge. Turns out, neither of us was on top of it.

On vacations like this, we usually leave one big backpack of diabetes stuff at the hotel. We repack the smaller diabetes go bag as needed. But "as needed" means someone has to know what's needed!

Luckily, we had a backup insulin pen and pen needles in the bag. That's one of my go-to items that has come in handy repeatedly over the years. I write the "no good" date on the pen and when it gets close, we pull the insulin out and use it in the pump. It's perfect if something goes wrong with the pump or the infusion set—or if you don't have a working set at all!

I was a little worried about calculating doses because I had no idea what his insulin-to-carb ratio was or his correction factor. Then I remembered we take photos now and then of his settings, so while they might not be up to the minute, they'd be close. But as I went to pull out my phone and scroll through my thousands of photos, Benny was a step ahead of me. "There's nothing wrong with my pump," he said. "We can use it as a calculator!"

That's what we did. We decided to not bolus again for breakfast; even though the site was leaking, we were about to walk a lot. We checked BG every two to three hours all day and gave shots as needed. It worked out just fine. We hadn't juggled tests strips and a meter in a long time, but it all came back. While it did not thrill Benny to take shots, he admitted it was better than missing a great day of rides and fun.

"Stacey," you may ask, "why was Benny having to use test strips to test blood sugar? He didn't have a pump infusion set, but didn't he still have his Dexcom on?"

Gentle reader, I forgot to mention that at that same breakfast, he also lost his phone. Somewhere in the confusion and excitement, Benny had put his phone down and never picked it back up. We were almost to the very first ride when he realized it. Of course, we ran back to the restaurant, but in just those ten minutes, it was gone.

In late 2017, when this story takes place, you could use the Tandem t:slim X2 pump as a Dexcom receiver. That update had become available just a few weeks earlier. I don't recall whether we didn't do that update or if we just didn't have that sensor info loaded into the pump. Hey, I don't write everything down! Either way, he was back to fingersticks.

Amazingly, we got the phone back! Universal told us to check with Lost and Found. I pinged the phone a few times, texting "THIS IS A MEDICAL DEVICE" hoping to shame or scare the person who took it into turning it in. I called Lost and Found every few hours and late the next day they had it! They said an employee found it in a different restaurant and immediately turned it in. So my guess is that the person who stole it saw the messages. Or they didn't realize how much of an out-of-date phone it was until later. Either way, that was a joyful day.

Diabetes complicates vacations outside of theme parks, of course, but we have found there is almost always a way to make it work. We went on two cruises with extended family when the children were young enough for the "kids' camp" programs. Benny always loved these. Lea was more lukewarm and preferred to stay with us. Our routine was to scope it out on the first day and see how comfortable the staff felt about watching a child with T1D.

In general, these camp programs will take kids with diabetes, but they won't care for them. In other words, your child will be responsible for checking BG and dosing. We brought Benny to the camp in between meals and planned to swing by if they gave the kids snacks or something else to eat. This got easier as he got a little older and could look at his Dexcom and treat lows. They're so active in those camps that high BG generally wasn't a problem for him!

We provided low treatments for these programs, simple stuff like tabs or gummies. Many of the cruise ships have strict protections in place for children with allergies, so check with them as the restrictions may go beyond peanuts or dairy. We're all trying to do the best we can for our children, so please be flexible on low treatments. If my child's favorite treatment for lows could be dangerous for another child, it's common sense for my kiddo to switch to a different treatment for one week.

One of my favorite stories of Benny in this kind of setting is the time he was about nine and went a little low. He had been eyeing the bar just outside the camp and he told the staff he was going to head there to get a drink. They let him go and he sat down at the bar and got some juice. (Of course, they should never have let him leave!) It was one of his coolest moments and happiest memories of that trip.

On another trip, we had the chance to go on a guided tour on horseback, something very out of the ordinary for my family! Benny was about eight years old; this was just a few months before we started using a CGM. I didn't want to scare the tour guide, but I wanted to let him know I might need to stop every so often for BG checks. The tour guide volunteered to take a Gatorade in his saddlebag and, of course, Benny and I had lots of other low stuff. Benny was in line right behind the guide and I was directly behind Benny. Lea and my mom and the rest of the party followed us. We had an incredible time! Of course, I asked Benny how he felt more than was probably necessary. We checked his BG via fingersticks at the breaks we took.

Years later, we were talking about the trip and Benny mentioned he never once thought he was behind the guide because of diabetes. He just thought he was lucky to be up front! I never really shared my planning with Benny until he was much older. I think that helped him to just jump in and enjoy, never realizing the safety net we'd stitched below him.

Because we've been able to navigate diabetes on all sorts of trips, it took me aback when a form I was filling out asked about any kind of medical condition that might "hamper" travel. What an odd way to word something.

We were celebrating my parents' fiftieth wedding anniversary. This was a trip that would involve snorkeling, swimming, and lots of sightseeing. Reading the form, I was afraid if I disclosed T1D they might not let Benny do anything!

I asked for advice from some more experienced diabetes moms I go to in situations like this. They all said disclose. You cannot hide it when you get there, and why would you want to? Better to find out what the story is ahead of time and either argue your case or find a Plan B to make sure the trip is still fun for Benny.

Here's what I wrote on social media:

> Update: I spoke with the tour people. They clarified that the form I had questions about was about mobility. They have apparently had situations where people show up in wheelchairs or need extra accommodations for walking. She encouraged me to leave T1D off the form and just tell the tour guide (if I want to) when we arrive. "You probably know a lot more about it than us. If you've traveled before and you're comfortable, that's completely up to you. Thanks for calling to check. We really appreciate that!"

Best outcome we could have hoped for! That was a terrific trip. We snorkeled almost every day. I bought a dry bag off Amazon and brought all the backup supplies with us on the boat every time. Those supplies included a meter and lancer, test strips, glucose tabs, and a protein bar. These were two- to three-hour tours very close to our primary base, so we decided not to bring any backup sensors or infusion sets. Easy enough to wait until we were back with the main group. I don't remember any problems with tech coming off; it may have happened, but it wasn't enough of an issue for me to note anywhere.

I spent a lot of time in the first book talking about my tips for travel. We've had all sorts of diabetes adventures on planes, in cars, and on boats! Travel with T1D takes a lot of preparation, packing, and patience. But it can be done! This time around, I want to share something we never did.

We've never asked for a disability pass. There are a lot of strong feelings about this in the community, so hear me out. I'm not holding that up as a good or a bad thing and my thinking on this matter has evolved over the years.

The first time we went to Disney World with Benny, he was about four years old. We spent an afternoon in the Magic Kingdom and then ate dinner and swam at the hotel. We went back the next morning as early as the park opened and had a splendid morning of rides and fun, with no long lines or waiting. It was brutal. The moon was still visible! That was a just quick taste, but it made me realize how important planning was if we wanted to do a longer trip.

We went back when the kids were seven and ten years old. By then, I'd heard about the Disability Access Service (DAS) pass, which differed greatly from what it is today. I believe it was basically a front-of-the-line pass. Slade and I talked about it, but we didn't feel it was necessary. Benny had lived with type 1 for five years by then and we'd never had an issue with waiting in lines or not being able to manage a situation. Also, we weren't going in the heat of the summer. Even without the pass, we had an amazing trip. And because of my bonkers Disney planning, we never waited over fifteen minutes for anything.

We've gone back to Disney World and Universal a few more times and we had season passes to our local amusement park, Carowinds, for many years. Our biggest diabetes issue was always about making sure we had supplies and who would carry them. I was basically the sherpa. When Benny got a little older, he carried a sling bag and usually shoved low stuff in his cargo shorts.

We honestly didn't think we needed a special pass, but, if I'm being honest, a big reason I was against it was because of how it had been presented to me on social media. "There's nothing good about diabetes except the front-of-the-line pass at Disney" is what I read online. "Our kids go through so much; they deserve this perk." It seemed less like a medical necessity and more like a consolation prize. That wasn't how we wanted Benny to look at his diabetes. A few years later, I started to see it differently.

In 2017, I went to the HealtheVoices conference, an event for advocates of different conditions and disabilities. I was sitting at a table of diabetes advocates when one woman said they were going to Disneyland and wanted to make sure we all knew about the disability passes. I volunteered that we didn't think we needed them and had never asked for one. She was surprised. We had a great and honest conversation where I admitted I thought of them as a perk we didn't need.

"But what if Benny actually does need it someday?" she asked.

She talked about all the reasons someone with diabetes might need the pass that have nothing to do with thinking about it as a reward. I'd already seen lots of examples of this—kids who really don't do well in the heat, others whose adrenaline spikes when they set foot in the parks due to all the excitement. We hadn't really had an issue, but by not educating Benny about his rights in this situation, I realized I might have left out something important.

Diabetes is a disability under the Americans with Disabilities Act. It entitles children to a 504 plan at school and accommodations during testing. Why did I look at this instance as something to avoid? Just because it was part of something fun? Benny and I have had some wonderful conversations about my thinking here. We've talked about how accommodations are there for a reason; they're not a reward. He seems to agree that he rarely needs a pass like this, but that he'll revisit it as he ventures out on his own.

The Disney DAS pass continues to change. Right now, it doesn't provide immediate access to experiences, but allows guests to request a return time for a specific experience that is comparable to the current standby wait. This means you don't have to wait physically in the line, but you have to wait out the time. You can register in advance, so be sure to check the website or Disney app before your visit.

Other parks have different policies. At Universal, many rides require you to store your bags in lockers. You can bring a small fanny pack or cross body bag on some rides, but there are a couple where they won't allow anything at all. For these, there are medical lockers much closer to the ride's loading area. Definitely scout this out in advance and ask staff while you're in line. We've used this with no issue.

As I'm writing this, I'm laughing at myself. Why would I think having access to the medical lockers is OK but using a DAS pass is not? I think it's because I could easily see the immediate need of a safe place to store our medical supplies. But really, it's splitting hairs.

At Carowinds and smaller parks, they often allow you to just place your bag on the side of the ride where you'll exit. You get into the ride vehicle, plop your bag on the platform and it's there when you get back. With medical stuff, most of us want more reassurance than that, which is why there are usually medical lockers. But I know when Benny goes without me, he'll just throw his bag wherever it's easy.

My biggest worry when I'm not with him is that he'll get stuck on a ride. When I was a teenager, my friends and I got stuck on Freefall at Great Adventure in New Jersey. Luckily, we weren't hanging at the top of the ride; we were already finished. We just had to wait a while to get off. I've drilled it into Benny to carry low stuff in his pockets. We've also talked about suspending his pump if he gets stuck somewhere and he's concerned about going low.

When Benny was little, we sought out the first aid areas or rest spots. Many parks have these for nursing moms or for families with special needs. It was a great place to do fingersticks, rehydrate, and take care of any issues. As he got older, we did those things more on the fly.

Our next big adventure is trying to visit all fifty states as a family. We have rules: feet on the ground outside, so connecting airports don't count, and we must get a photo of all four of us. We're up to twenty-nine states as of this writing. The biggest obstacle to completing our quest will be getting everyone together—between college and work, my children aren't available like they were when they were younger! It's wild to note that the challenge to travel here isn't diabetes.

As I've talked to international and adventure travelers for my podcast, they've all said the same thing. You can have highs and lows with diabetes wherever you are. Why let that keep you stuck at home? Go see the world! It's a fabulous attitude and one I try to emulate.

ASK YOUR DOCTOR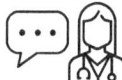

■ What supplies do I need for this trip?

■ Do I need a doctor's note for travel?

■ Can you write a prescription or give us samples, so we have backup supplies for our trip?

■ I use an insulin pump. Should I get a backup prescription for long-acting insulin?

■ I use vials for my insulin pump. Do you recommend backup pens for travel?

“ Most people end up loving whatever pump system they choose—as much as you can love a medical device! ”

CHAPTER 10

Choosing an Insulin Pump

B enny started using an insulin pump six months after diagnosis. We were worried about how a two-year-old would react to being attached to something 24-7, but he did great. OK, the first time we showed it to him, he threw it across the floor! But after we explained a little bit more about it and had him wear it without insulin for a day, he was good to go. I was stunned that my rambunctious toddler never tried to mess with the buttons or pull off the pump.

We have always used a tubed pump, first the Animas models and now the Tandem t:slim X2. Benny has selected his own technology for a long time now and he's always elected to stay with the tubes.

How did we make that initial choice? It wasn't easy. It's hard to believe, but in 2006, there were more choices in the US for pumps. We sat down with our educator and went through the options. I finally asked her to show me the one she thought was the best combination of simplicity and ease of use and would accomplish our goals of flexibility and precision in dosing. I think what I said was, "Give me the idiotproof one!"

There are countless Facebook posts about "which pump should I get?" and we've done several podcast episodes about this. The good thing—and what makes the choice difficult—is that they're all just fine. There are pros and cons to each system, so it largely comes down to personal preference.

For about the last five years, there have only been three main choices of pump technology in the United States. As I'm writing this chapter, there are two additional systems in front of the US Food and Drug Administration (FDA) and at least two more in the pipeline. I'll touch on each here, but I don't want to do a deep dive as each system will probably have changes and improvements by the time you're reading this. What doesn't change are the questions to ask yourself when you think about which pump may be best for your child. I'll try to go through some of the most important to us; of course, your medical team needs to be involved in these decisions as all pumps are prescription items in the United States.

Do we want to switch to a pump at all?

Social media might make it seem like no one is one using MDI anymore, but that's hardly the case. According to the T1D Exchange Quality Improvement Collaborative, about 60 percent of children with type 1 in the United States use an insulin pump.[13] If you decide to stay with shots, there are great newer options there too. Smart pens and apps make it a lot easier to keep track of dosing. The InPen and Bigfoot Biomedical systems even recommend dosing.

What's available?

There are three insulin pump companies making systems that are FDA approved and commercially available in the United States as of this writing: Medtronic, Tandem Diabetes Care, and Insulet Corporation. You can use all three as a stand-alone insulin pump or as part of an automated insulin delivery (AID) system. Put simply, an AID system is made up of the insulin pump, a software program or algorithm within the pump, and a continuous glucose monitor (CGM). Those three elements work together to automate insulin delivery to improve Time in Range.

AID is a more recent term for what used to be called hybrid closed-loop, artificial pancreas, predictive insulin suspension, etc.

There is no commercial system out yet or in front of the FDA that is completely automated. With all of these systems, the user must still manually give insulin doses for food and/or some corrections.

We shorthand these systems a lot, and it can be confusing. For example, "Control-IQ" in conversation, means the Tandem t:slim X2 pump, with the Control-IQ software and a Dexcom G6 CGM. If someone is using "Omnipod 5" it means they're wearing an Insulet Omnipod 5 Pod, with the Omnipod 5 software and a Dexcom G6 CGM. Medtronic has a few systems out there, but as of this writing, the newest in the US is the Medtronic MiniMed 770G pump, with SmartGuard software, and the Guardian Sensor 3 CGM.

There are three more systems in front of the FDA right now: Medtronic's MiniMed 780G, Tidepool Loop, and the iLet Bionic Pancreas from Beta Bionics. There are at least two other pump systems looking to get US approval in the next two years, including Ypsomed and Sigi.

You'll notice later that I don't include the question "What pump should I get?" in this chapter's "ASK YOUR DOCTOR" section. While most endocrinologists and health care providers don't play favorites, I have heard of many cases where they are well-versed in one pump system and reluctant to learn another. Each pump system also has its own data-download link for health-care providers to use. If a small doctor's office has invested in one bit of hardware, they may not have the budget for another. Just something to be aware of and ask about if your endo won't give you options.

What's the difference between tubed and tubeless?

When we talk about insulin pumps, there are two types: tubed and tubeless. Both are a small mechanical device, a little larger than a pager, worn outside the body. Both deliver insulin through a small cannula under the skin and that cannula is inserted with a needle. In most cases, the needle goes in, then comes out and leaves the cannula behind a few millimeters below the skin.

With a tubed pump, there are auto inserters, most of which are spring-loaded and require a button push or a squeeze to activate. For the very brave, there are manual inserters, which is exactly as it sounds—you push the needle in by hand. Most infusion sets are meant to stay in place for two to three days, and then you insert a new one in a different location. The pump delivers the insulin through a thin, flexible plastic tube—anywhere from twenty-four to forty-eight inches long—that attaches to the infusion set.

Tandem and Medtronic pumps are tubed. Medtronic has just come out with a longer-lasting, seven-day infusion set. It's getting good reports in real-world studies but seems to be in very limited release. I don't know anyone yet who's used it, but we're keeping an eye on it!

The tubeless pump is also referred to as a patch pump or a pod. With this type, the mechanisms are very similar, but everything is in one piece. The cannula is still inserted under the skin with a needle, but there is no long tubing to connect the pump to the infusion set. The inserter, the cannula, and the insulin cartridge are all together, and the whole thing sits on the skin.

Right now, Insulet's Omnipod is the only tubeless pump in the US approved for T1D. It has an external controller you need to carry; tubed pumps are operated by buttons or a touch screen on the pump itself. All of these systems are moving toward, or already have, smartphone control.

I am thrilled by the move toward additional phone control. As a parent of a young child on a pump, the best added feature we got was what they called the "meter remote." Animas added that a few years after Benny started using it, so he was about six when we got it. It's so much easier to dose insulin from a little remote rather than dig out the pump when your child is sleeping, or in a car seat, or playing nearby. When Animas went out of business, we lost that feature. Tandem now has its own bolus by phone feature, so we've got it back.

What does my insurance cover?

In the US, this must be one of the first questions you ask. Over the years, I've learned that the best people to talk to about coverage often aren't the people at your health insurance company, but the people at the pump companies. They all have a staff dedicated to what's called verification of benefits. You will still need a prescription and you'll probably have to talk to your insurer at least once, but the pump companies can get you started in this process very quickly. That makes sense; you're going to need not just the pump, but the ongoing supplies. They have a vested interest in making sure you're covered.

It's worth asking about pharmacy coverage versus what's called Durable Medical Equipment (DME) coverage. This can change depending on the agreement between your pump company and your insurer. Sometimes you can use either and often one is cheaper. Sometimes you're locked in with few options. Often insurers will limit you to one insulin pump under DME coverage every four years. Find out as much as you can before you decide.

What problem am I trying to solve?
What am I trying to improve in our diabetes care?

We knew why we were switching to a pump: we wanted to have more flexibility and accuracy in dosing. After the first two weeks home from the hospital, Benny didn't mind taking shots. We weren't switching because of that. It was the dosing; he was two years old and he needed teeny tiny wisps of insulin. We were trying to measure out quarter-unit doses with syringes that weren't marked that way. Insulin pens didn't come in half units at that time, and they wouldn't have helped us much if they did! Once I learned a pump could dose at 0.025 units, I knew it would help us be more accurate.

AID systems are another terrific reason to switch; once I found out they can make up to 300 dosing decisions a day, I was in awe. No wonder we were far from perfect in our management! A computer can do a much better job as an almost-pancreas than a person.

If you're not sure what your reason is, other than it seems like every other kid has a pump, it's worth taking some time to think it through.

What's your routine, and what do you carry with you?

There are practical issues to think about. Some people carry a backpack or handbag wherever they go and love to have a bag with lots of pockets to organize things. Others want to travel as lightly as possible.

Some kids seem to lose things every time they turn around. You laugh, but this was a big reason we didn't consider Omnipod when Benny was younger. There was no chance of him not leaving the controller device at school or on the bus or at a friend's house. As these systems move to phone control, this is less of an issue, but it's still worth thinking about.

How does it feel?

You've probably heard that tubing gets caught on doorknobs and that pods get smacked off in doorways or during sports. That's all true. But I think most people get used to whatever technology they wear and figure out how to manage it. We know children and adults who, over the years, have worn just about every pump available. Most say it's like getting used to wearing a new ring or a watch. The first day you put it on, it feels strange, but if you wear it every day, your body gets used to it.

We saw this in action when we started potty training. We did this one month after starting the pump, because why not create all sorts of chaos all at once?! Benny wore his infusion set on his backside, so part of the process included making sure he knew to be careful taking his pants on and off.

From my blog in August 2007:

> The pump is attached to his body by a thin tube attached to what we call a "button" on his bottom, the infusion set. We've discovered a unique problem with that. When a two-year-old tries to take off his own pants, he can pull the button out. He's done it three times already. Because of that, he's now pretty cautious. Anytime we go to the potty, he tells me, "Be careful my button!"[14]

We lost a few sets, but with the passing of time, it just became a habit. Thank goodness for elastic-waist toddler pants!

Ask your educator to physically show you the options. Besides size and tubes, you may want to listen to the noises the pump makes and observe how well you can see the screen. It's hard to get the feel for these devices without literally touching them. As Benny got older, we looked at switching to pods, but he felt it was too bulky under clothes. Other friends from diabetes camp had the opposite reaction; they didn't like the idea of tubing.

I think it's worth mentioning that both types of pumps and all three brands I've mentioned are used by professional athletes. To me, that shows that they all work for rambunctious and super-active kids. It's less of a matter of wear and tear and more about preference.

Should I wait for the next model, even if it means coming out of warranty?

This is a tough one, but I vote no.

OK, that's too quick. What I mean is quite often the marketing departments of these companies get a little ahead of their engineering—or at least, ahead of the FDA. They may have announced a long pipeline of cool devices, but that doesn't mean any of it will be available anytime soon. A good example is that when I wrote the first book in 2019, all three pump companies were promising new AID systems. Then the pandemic hit.

Tandem got Control-IQ approved in January 2020, but Omnipod 5 approval was delayed until 2022. Medtronic's MiniMed 780G was approved in Europe in 2020 but is still under FDA review as of this writing.

I'm also very uncomfortable letting Benny's pump go out of warranty. I don't really care if my refrigerator warranty runs out, but we don't take chances with medical devices. In the sixteen years Benny's been pumping, we've had two instances where we needed a new pump. In both cases, we had a new one in hand and were pumping again within twenty-four hours. That's reassuring to me.

However you feel about warranties, please be careful about buying now on future promises. I hate to say it, but we've received some bad information and over-promises from well-meaning (I hope) company salespeople. We've learned that unless there is a launch date from the company that you can see on their website or has appeared in an email directly to you, you can't rely on verbal promises.

Where can I get more information?

DiabetesWise is a great resource that I've come across more recently. This is an initiative from Stanford University School of Medicine, staff and faculty there, and people living with diabetes. It's independently funded, so it's not beholden to any device company or manufacturer. At www.diabeteswise.org, they have information on all the current systems. You're able to put in your personal preferences to see what might best suit your needs. This year they added DiabetesWise Pro to help providers keep up on all the changes.

What about DIY?

The Do-It-Yourself diabetes community, also known as the #WeAreNotWaiting community, could be its own book! This is an amazing, loose-knit group that started pushing years ago to see what improvements they could make to the communication between insulin pumps and CGMs. Tired of waiting for commercial systems to catch up to what these very smart people knew was possible, they jumped in. Nightscout, CGM in the Cloud, OpenAPS, RileyLink, and "looping" are some terms you may be familiar with. These are all thanks to the Do-It-Yourself community.

I have a lot of respect and affection for these folks, but I will not go in-depth on these systems here. First, we have used none of them, so I'm hardly an expert. But more importantly, they can change and improve faster than the commercial systems, as they are not FDA approved or commercially available, so anything I'd say could become dated almost immediately. I will say that I firmly believe what we're seeing from the pump and CGM companies has been pushed along by the DIY folks. They showed it was possible, it was safe, and that there was demand.

If you'd like to learn more, I have a bunch of podcast episodes featuring these amazing people. You can search for "WeAreNotWaiting" (all one word) in the search box at www.diabetes-connections.com. Or just search that hashtag on social media.

What if we hate it? What if we mess it up?

Remember, a pump isn't something that's permanent; it's not implanted. If your child really hates it or it's not working out how you hoped, you can take it off and try again later. Or you can work with your endocrinologist to switch to a new system as soon as your insurance allows, or sooner if you can argue medical necessity.

Most people end up loving whatever system they choose—as much as you can love a medical device! But these are very personal items; people with diabetes wear them 24-7. We did an episode where I asked my listeners to weigh in; I asked for fans of whatever system they used to tell us what they liked. That episode should be pretty reassuring. All three of the systems I mentioned had people singing the praises of the technology.

No matter which pump you choose, you will make mistakes in use, technology will fail occasionally, and you'll forget supplies here and there along the way. Take photos of pump settings with your phone or write them down anytime they change. Make sure you have backup supplies, like syringes or pen needles, in case you need to go back to shots. Using a pump is far from foolproof and it's always a good idea to have a backup plan.

How much should I involve my child in this choice?

I'm putting this question last because I know some have very strong feelings about this being solely a parental decision. I feel completely the opposite way. Once your child is old enough to understand, they should have a say in their diabetes technology. As I've said, there are two things over which people with diabetes have no choice: insulin must go in and blood glucose numbers must be checked. After that, there are a lot of variables, one of which is using an insulin pump and another is which type.

We made those decisions for Benny at age two, but I think age six or seven, depending on your child, is a great time to include them in these decisions. You may have your heart set on a pump you saw on a friend's child or on Instagram, but if your tween is set on something else, please remember that they are the one who'll wear it. And if your child wants to stay with shots and your endo says they are safe and happy, please consider and respect their feelings.

ASK YOUR DOCTOR

- How would an insulin pump benefit my child's diabetes management?

- Taking my child's age and our experience into account, what are some factors you'd recommend we look for in an insulin pump system?

- Does your office offer a class or meeting where we can see all our options for pumps?

- Will you help us navigate with our insurer or appeal if they don't cover the pump we choose?

" There is no moral value in how much insulin your child uses. Repeat that. Write it out and tape it on the bathroom mirror if you need to. There is nothing 'good' about using less insulin or 'bad' about using more. **"**

CHAPTER 11

Going Untethered

I started the *Diabetes Connections* podcast when Benny was ten years old. If you go back and listen to those early episodes, you can hear how scared I was of the teen years. I was terrified that he'd rebel or stop doing simple diabetes tasks or resent us in some way. I had no idea that the real problem for us would be massive insulin resistance.

Most people increase their insulin dosing during puberty. There are a lot of reasons for that. Hormones such as testosterone and estrogen work against insulin, as do stress hormones like cortisol. A lot of kids get markedly hungrier during puberty and, of course, they're growing a lot too. Add on their natural increased desire for more independence and it's a wild time.

When Benny was eleven and in sixth grade, he had his highest A1C since diagnosis. I knew it would be on the high side, but I was still shocked. I'm not proud of my reaction; I burst into tears! I usually try to stay calm in front of the kids, but this seemed awful. Was the endo going to yell at me? Or give Benny a stern lecture?

Dr. V laughed. "Welcome to puberty," he said to Benny. "Don't worry about your mom. She's going to be just fine. This is part of the process." He took out the pump and cranked up all the settings. Dr. V explained that while Benny was still a tween, his body was already acting like a teen's body, and it was nothing to be alarmed by. He explained that kids start puberty at different ages. We just know about the T1D kids because of their noticeable insulin resistance. He added that Benny's insulin needs would most likely go back down when he came out of puberty.

That all made sense to me and helped me feel better. But what still frustrated me was that we had changed nothing. Benny was still checking and dosing. He wasn't hiding diabetes; he wasn't angry about it. Benny wasn't perfect, but we'd never asked him to be. This wasn't about a change in behavior or attitude. It was about a tremendous change in his body that he couldn't control—that I couldn't control.

It's hard to overstate how big these changes were and how quickly they seemed to happen. Remember, Benny was diagnosed at twenty-three months. I vividly remember trying to draw up a quarter unit of insulin in a syringe only marked to half units. When we switched to an insulin pump, his hourly basal rate was 0.025 units. We chose that first pump because it could dose in units that tiny. To watch that tick up to one full unit was dramatic—or so I thought.

Benny's basal rate doubled from age eleven to twelve. It doubled again by age thirteen. We were just pouring insulin into that kid! Lots of people say "they need what they need," and that's true; if Benny didn't have diabetes, his pancreas would just naturally be pumping out elephant-sized doses of insulin.

There is no moral value in how much insulin you or your child uses. Repeat that. Write it out and tape it on the bathroom mirror if you need to. There is nothing "good" about using less insulin or "bad" about using more. It's about using what you and your health team determine is right for your child.

I was shocked to find out not everyone on our health team understood that. Here's a Facebook post from 2015:

Just gave the nurse at our endo an earful. Need an insulin refill—we have the mail order, ninety-day supply thing and they haven't increased his prescription since cranking up the basal last year. She said to me, "He's only twelve. Why does he need so much insulin?" I was very, very nice (I promise) but after answering her question—because his daily total basal doubled in eighteen months—I told her that was not the best way to ask that question. I pointed out she immediately put me on the defensive when I'm sure she didn't mean to. She was really apologetic, and we had a nice discussion about it. But OMG! My kid can't be the only tween with a teenage body (as my endo says), right? Give me the insulin!!

We soon hit another roadblock. Even after getting all the insulin and doing all the doses, something still wasn't right. His blood sugar was staying higher longer. You've heard others say this, but it seemed like the insulin was just water.

Was it the infusion set? Maybe a longer cannula might work better? We tried that for about three weeks, but it didn't make a difference. We were still getting maybe two days out of each infusion set when they're meant to last for three. The cannula wasn't bent, but they just did not work as they had for the previous decade. Half the time, Benny would dose on day two and insulin would leak out down his stomach!

Benny was getting frustrated with all the site changes and cartridge refills. I was getting frustrated with how nothing we did seemed to work. I didn't want my son, who was willing to put in the effort, to get burned out because he wasn't seeing results! Finally, I turned to my community. Of course, another D-Mom had the answer for us. Thank you, Cheryl, for suggesting we go untethered.

Untethered means making use of an insulin pump while also taking an injection of long-acting insulin. As far as I can tell, Dr. Steven Edelman, who lives with type 1 himself, coined the term back in 2004.[15]

Some people use the word "untethered" to mean that they only use the pump for boluses and all basal comes from the long-acting insulin. It's also referred to as POLI or Pumping On Long-Acting Insulin. For our purposes here, I'm going to use the terms interchangeably to mean using some basal from a shot and some basal and all boluses from the pump, but it's important to note there are a few ways to skin this cat. You always want to ask your health care team for advice before doing so.

I had heard about untethered for years, but it seemed odd to me. Why would you go through all the bother that is an insulin pump—the insertions, wearing the pump itself, schlepping the separate controller if you've got a Pod—and then add a daily shot? I would soon find the answer: it works!

Dr. V thought it was worth a try. We started with 30 percent basal from that daily shot and 70 percent basal and all boluses from the pump. We saw an improvement right away! Over about two months, we adjusted dosing until it was 50–50 percent from shot and pump, which worked amazingly well.

I was trying to remember exactly how and when we started. I was able to triangulate using my Facebook posts and my Google calendar. It was October 2018, right after an overnight school field trip. I wanted to wait two more weeks because I was out of town two weekends in a row and Benny didn't want to start on a school day. Of course, after all that planning, Benny and my husband decided to just go for it while I was away! They're a great team, so I was only a little worried.

I'm so glad they didn't wait! It was incredible. Once those basal rates in the pump came down, everything seemed to work so much more efficiently. He wasn't having to refill cartridges and do site changes as often, which was his chief concern. His Time in Range and A1C levels came back to pre-puberty numbers, which was my primary concern.

I couldn't find any studies or medical literature to back this up, but it's my belief that pump infusion sets get overloaded when you try to push very large individual or daily doses through them. That's just not what they're designed for. We changed nothing else but adding that daily long-acting and it made an enormous difference.

Once I started researching untethered, I learned it wasn't only a benefit for teenagers who are overloading their infusion sets. In fact, most people who show up in blogs and medical journals for untethered are adults.

I spoke to a few people who use this method, and a few told me they had trouble, especially at first, trusting an insulin pump. That makes sense to me, especially for people who've used shots every day since diagnosis. With a pump, not only do you have to trust the technology, but you don't physically see the insulin going in as you do with a shot. One person told me she wanted to make sure the pump system was working, that untethered helped her ease into the process. She stopped untethered after a couple of months. Another person I spoke to had the same concerns and has stayed on untethered because it's working so well for her.

I have another friend who shared that she worried about everything that could go wrong with her insulin pump. This went beyond concerns about switching over; she was having trouble sleeping and found herself checking her pump all day long to make sure it was working. Her endocrinologist prescribed untethered to help her with that anxiety. It's made a tremendous difference for her too.

Untethered is also an option during the summer months, or anytime you might be in the water a lot. It's convenient to take off the insulin pump while you're at the beach and only reconnect for snacks and meals. You don't have to worry as much about missed basal or about sand in your pump!

Whatever the reason, I think it's important to know this is an option and that it's one you can use for however long you wish. Benny stayed with untethered for two years. By the time he was fifteen, his insulin needs had come back down. We had also started Control-IQ which made a difference in how much insulin he used.

If you start, it's a good idea to keep additional basal rate profiles in the insulin pump. We had "untethered" and "pump-only" setups. It's a lot easier to switch back and forth that way.

You can do untethered with any long-acting insulin brand, but our endocrinologist recommended a newer type called Tresiba. When I describe it, I always feel like I'm talking about whiskey! It's smooth. There's no burn. It's very steady.

That's all true, but Tresiba is a bit different from Lantus or Levemir. It lasts longer in the body, which worked very well for Benny. It takes about three to five days before you reach a steady state. After that, there's a little more flexibility in when you must take it. Ask your doctor, but if you miss the dose of Tresiba, we were told it's OK to take it at least eight hours before the next dose. That's such a great safety net! Benny was terrific about remembering to take Tresiba every day, but it was great to know he had some grace for the times he forgot.

Of course, like everything diabetes, you're at the mercy of insurance. We were lucky that Tresiba was covered for us; at the time, all insurers did not cover a much newer long-acting. Again, you can use any long-acting with untethered, so check what's covered in your plan.

If you check the dates and read this book carefully, you'll know that we started untethered right around the same time we started Basal-IQ, the software from Tandem that allowed the pump to automatically cut off insulin when blood glucose went below 80. We talked with our endo and educator about how that might affect the new routine and kept going with both. We had to be careful about treating lows; the pump system had no way of knowing Benny was also taking long-acting. But since we were much more concerned with Benny's higher BGs, we thought it would work out fine. It did.

In January 2020 we switched to Control-IQ, the automated insulin system (AID) from Tandem. Again, we debated coming off untethered, but decided to keep going and see how it worked. Again, it was great. We probably had to pay more attention to the AID system than most, but it still worked very well. After a few months, the combination of the efficiency of the AID system and Benny's natural insulin needs coming down eased us into transitioning out of untethered.

We had one big mix-up with Tresiba and it was long after we had stopped untethered. Benny was at a sleepover and forgot to charge his pump. It was very late and so, rather than wait for his pump to recharge, he gave himself a dose of long-acting, which he had in his bag. To his teen brain, that made sense. It was almost the right thing to do. As I mentioned, it can take three to five days for Tresiba to reach a steady state in the body, so that late-night dose probably showed up at least a day or so later. He plugged his pump in and it started giving him a basal a short time later. I complimented him on his attempt at problem-solving even as I wanted to smack him for letting the pump run down. Oh, teens!

Honestly, I give Benny so much credit. He rolls his eyes at me when I try to tell him I'm proud, but it was no fun to take a shot every day, especially on top of all the other aspects of diabetes management! It was a terrific way to manage a tough time.

Not everyone needs to do this, of course. But if your tween or teen's blood sugar is high all the time, if they're tired of changing Pods or infusion sets every two days, going untethered may be something to think about.

ASK YOUR DOCTOR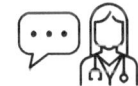

- Are you familiar with untethered or POLI methods? Is this something you'd recommend for us?

- What long-acting insulin would you recommend we use?

- What ratio of long-acting basal and pump basal would you recommend we start with?

He must really struggle, right? If his numbers are 'good,' why wouldn't I just share everything? There are lots of reasons to keep our information private; I promise, it has nothing to do with terrible diabetes management. Remember, I'm the Worst; Benny is doing just fine.

CHAPTER 12

The Numbers Game

When Benny was about nine or ten, a well-meaning staff member at camp asked him what his A1C was. This was at "regular" non-diabetes camp, and they were giving out ice cream to the kids. I wasn't there, of course, and when Benny relayed the story to me later, he explained he did not know what to say. He did what made sense to him: walked away and found someone else to give him the ice cream. Smart kid!

My son's A1C should not have been a means test to whether he could eat ice cream. I talked to the camp about that, but part of going to a non-diabetes program means learning to deal with people who aren't quite as educated about diabetes. Benny was getting very good at managing that skill and it's served him well all these years later.

I think he was also well served by not knowing his A1C. Let me explain. Because I've made much of our diabetes story public, I'm often asked about Benny's numbers. It surprises most people to hear that we don't share them. In an age where people post photos of their kids posing with their A1Cs on cute signs, and even work their numbers into social media handles and hashtags, why don't I post about my kid's diabetes digits?

He must really struggle, right? If his numbers are "good," why wouldn't I just share everything? There are lots of reasons to keep our information private; I promise, it has nothing to do with terrible diabetes management. Remember, I'm the Worst; Benny is doing just fine.

I shared more information about Benny when he was younger, but things were a bit different back then. Hard to remember, but social media wasn't as big back in 2006. The iPhone had just come out and we were just learning about photo sharing and even how to talk on social media. I'm considered an early adopter because I joined Twitter and Facebook in 2008!

I shared a lot of specific numbers, including A1Cs. Just about every time we went to the endocrinologist, I would post about the experience and talk about how Benny was doing. Of course, that meant posting photos of his meter (no CGM screenshots yet!) and sharing his labs. I kept that up for a few years, but then I became friends with Moira McCarthy, who is a well-known author, writer, and diabetes advocate. You can hear her as my cohost of the *Ask the D-Moms* episodes on the podcast.

Moira asked me to think about why I was sharing so much. I remember feeling incredibly defensive. Why wouldn't I share? It seemed like everyone else did! What could hurt about sharing what, at the time, I called "our" numbers? But I took a step back and stopped posting while I processed what she was getting at. I never started posting numbers again.

Moira's point is that no matter what the A1C number is, when we share it, we're placing judgment on the parent, or the child, or the adult with diabetes. Here's what Moira wrote on her blog, over ten years ago. It's brilliant advice that might be even more relevant today.

I think we, as a diabetes community, are a bit messed up when it comes to how we discuss, share, and yes, *wield* our a1C. Be it our own or that of our children, a1C's somehow feel like judgments. Heck: sometimes they feel like sentences.

Sometimes—most times—the a1C results feel like a report card.

And I would go as far as to say this is not because a high or low a1C is good or bad; it's because we wrap our entire "diabetes being" up in that number. I wish we could change that.

First, off, I'm not telling you an a1C is not an important measure of how things are going for the person with diabetes. It absolutely is. There is no doubt (and study after study after study proves) that a lower-range a1C is just plain better for a person with diabetes. That's not what I'm talking about at all. What I'm talking about is how we share it as a community, toss it around at one another and hold it up like a trophy when we can.

I don't think that's good. In fact, I'd go as far as to say I'd love a diabetes world where everyone just kept their a1C's to themselves, other than extremely private conversations.[16]

Moira advocates treating an A1C like what it is: a lab number. We don't commonly share our cholesterol numbers or blood pressure readings, right? Moira pushed me to share more about our lives with diabetes, to talk about what felt good and what we struggled with. It made sense to me, and I've done it ever since.

I think I was already primed for this advice because of my radio career. Stay with me on this. I promise it'll make sense! I worked in radio for a very long time. While I was in college, I started my career working as the weekend reporter at WSYR, the NewsTalk station in Syracuse, New York. After college, I was a local TV anchor and reporter for many years and then returned to radio, hosting the morning show at WBT in Charlotte, North Carolina.

My program director at WBT, Bill White, used to caution us against putting too much stock into the ratings. As you likely know, ratings measure how many people are listening. That's not just for bragging rights; it sets the commercial rates. Salespeople use the ratings to sell advertising on a station, and that helps pay everyone's salaries.

WBT never really sold on those numbers strictly, though, because we had a very desirable audience. Our audience was older, with more money, and a lot of loyalty to the station. We didn't have to live and die by the ratings; we could sell on the value of the audience.

That's a fantastic place to be for a NewsTalk station. Think about when you might listen to all-news radio, if you listen at all these days. You'd want it when there's a power failure or a local emergency. Live and local radio is an incredible medium for in-the-moment news; in terms of traditional media, it can't be beat for immediacy. We'd see huge rating spikes when breaking news events would happen and large drop-offs when there weren't exciting stories going on.

If we started taking those numbers personally, it would be easy to feel flattered and triumphant when the ratings went up, and just as easy to feel deflated and defeated when they went down. It's fun to imagine you're the reason the morning show was number one in the market that quarter. It's a horrible feeling to have anyone believe your poor performance is responsible for the ranking to slump.

Our program director knew about the fragile egos of radio "talent" and he was smart to caution us against riding that up-and-down cycle. He told us the best thing we could do was focus on serving our listeners well and putting out the best show we could every day. He didn't want us to get our egos wrapped up in the highs and lows. You see where I'm going with this and diabetes, right?

Of course, numbers are important, more so in diabetes than in radio! Of course, we need to pay attention to them, but we can't run our lives around them. We can't let them have the emotional power that many seem to want to give them. I've been guilty of this too. But once you realize the numbers are information and guidelines with no moral value, I can't tell you how freeing it is. Your value as a parent does not come from your child's A1C. It is *not* your report card. It's not your child's report card either.

Our kids absorb all of this. They may not know their exact A1C, but they know if you put a lot of stock in it. I'm seeing more parents posting photos of their kids with cute signs showing their numbers. That's awesome when your five-year-old looks adorable, with a little handwritten sign that says, "A1C 6.7!" But what happens when your eleven-year-old notices you don't want to post about her 7.9 or her 8.5? These kids are very perceptive; they know we're sharing their numbers and they know there's a judgment being made.

There is another incredibly important reason to think twice before posting all these numbers. If nothing I've said resonates with you, maybe this will: you're making a choice to leave a trail of your child's health information on the internet. Nothing online is private. Not a closed Facebook group, not an Instagram story, not a Twitter post. There are already instances of advertisers, health care companies, and others buying access to health information online, particularly on Facebook.

The market in medical records is huge—estimated at $13.5 billion annually.[17] Artificial intelligence can now cross-reference data in powerful new ways. One of the worst outcomes of this, in my opinion, is that patients are being denied care or insurance coverage based on information payers drew from their social media activities after combining datasets to reidentify them. There are quite a few groups trying to fight this. A good one is a patient group called the Light Collective, if you'd like to learn more.

The more I learn about how much online privacy isn't private at all, the more I'm convinced not posting these numbers is the way to go. It's reinforced my reluctance to share them all these years, even for the times when I really want to brag!

There is another school of thought that you don't even need to tell younger children what their A1C is. As I said earlier, Benny didn't know his A1C for many years, probably not until high school, because it wasn't something we stressed. But we always talked about it in front of him. These days, more endocrinologists are just writing it down for the parents or emailing it through a health portal. The latter is great because it's protected by the Health

Insurance Portability and Accountability Act (HIPAA) in a way that Facebook obviously is not.

Recently, there's been a move away from A1C as the only measure of diabetes management and toward what's called Time in Range (TIR). This is due to the rise of CGM adoption, and it gives a more complete picture of blood glucose. After all, you can have a lower A1C and still have plenty of high readings, if you also have a lot of very low ones. The "range" in Time in Range is generally accepted to be 70–180 and the goal for most people is 70 percent. I agree that TIR is a much better and more useful measurement. But again, it's a number and if we can measure it, we will compare it. That's just human nature. We need to be just as careful about throwing around our child's TIR as we do the A1C.

Are there ever times when it's OK to post any numbers? It may surprise you that I'll say yes. In context, when you have specific community questions or need some support, it's helpful to share an A1C or another number. It's the mindless, automatic sharing I'm cautioning against here. The every-quarter post of the A1C. The snapshot of the latest straight-line graph. Not a question about "Am I all alone with this?" situation or "We're struggling with this" situation. I'm still very reluctant to share Benny's information, but I can see some situations where it would make sense, again to add context and to ask questions, not to simply throw out there because I have that information in front of me.

And, if this isn't clear, I'm 100 percent in favor of sharing numbers with your actual friends and family if you have questions or need support. Within the small of group of D-Moms and women with type 1 that I call my in-real-life and not just social media friends, I have shared many numbers over the years.

I will never forget when Benny had his highest A1C since diagnosis. That week I was lucky enough to be part of a local conference where a bunch of us stayed for late-night schmoozing, drinks, and heartfelt talk. I shared our situation and my feelings of helplessness and failure. They buoyed and reassured me; I left feeling stronger, unashamed, and no longer alone. Had I shared that number on social media, I don't think I would have received the same amount of support. I would have opened myself up to judgment from people I don't know. Worse, that number would still be out there for insurers or just nasty people to find.

How do we talk about diabetes overall if we don't celebrate or share numbers? It's hard to do, I know. But I would encourage you to look at other milestones. The victories for me were the adventures with grandparents, bedtime snuggles, even milestones like potty training and learning to read. For older kids, maybe it's participating in sports or the school play or (heaven help me) getting their driver's permit. Even if diabetes management isn't "perfect," it's tough to accomplish those goals and feel good about them if diabetes is completely out of whack. Celebrate that hard work.

I urge you to try this. You may find it incredibly freeing not to share your numbers, not to share your child's numbers. Our children are so much more than their A1C or their TIR or the last twenty-four hours on a graph, and we've got to stop defining them in that way. After all, we're not raising numbers; we're raising children.

ASK YOUR DOCTOR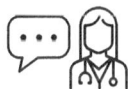

- Is there a portal or another private way to communicate my child's lab results and information?

- Do you look at Time in Range as well as the A1C? What target range do you recommend for my child's age and stage of diabetes?

- There is so much information in diabetes. How do your patients who thrive with T1D make sense of it all?

" The problem with telling your kids 'Diabetes can't stop you' is that they come to believe it! Kidding, a bit, but not entirely. How could we tell Benny that he was being responsible and independent and then not follow up? "

CHAPTER 13

The Trip to Israel—the Plan

This was my most popular tweet of 2021:

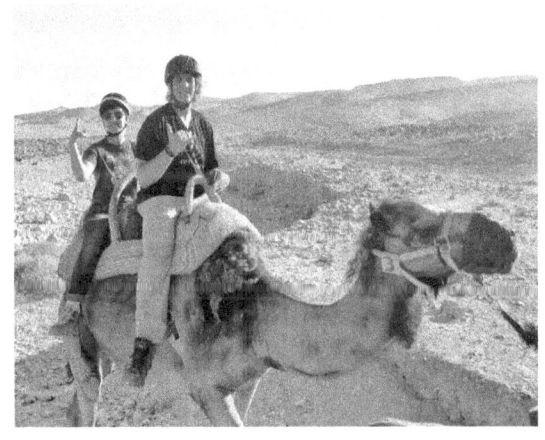

This week on the podcast . . .
Benny: "It was amazing! Thanks for letting me go!"
Stacey: "I wanted to puke. What was I thinking?"
#DiabetesParenting my friends.

This is probably my biggest flex so far as a diabetes parent. I still can't believe we did it. In 2021, Benny spent one month in Israel with a non-diabetes camp program while we stayed home, an ocean away.

As I've mentioned before, camp is a huge part of my family's tradition. My dad went, my sister and I both went, and so did my husband. Different camps, but all for several weeks, every summer. My daughter started sleepaway camp at age nine, so when Benny neared that age, he wanted to go as well.

I did an entire chapter on summer camp (diabetes and "regular") in the first book, so I won't rehash everything here. I will say that having Benny go to a diabetes sleepaway camp for one week at age seven made me a feel a little better about sending him to the regular camp the next year. He did both every summer until he was fifteen, when he chose to stop going to D-Camp.

I knew for years we were building toward this trip. The summer after sophomore year in high school, this group goes to Israel. They don't even have a regular camp session. There are lots of options for kids who don't go to Israel; my daughter went to a leadership program in New York, for example. But Benny knew early on that he wanted to be part of the Israel trip, and he reminded us every year.

The problem with telling your kids "Diabetes can't stop you" is that they come to believe it! Kidding, a bit, but not entirely. How could we tell Benny that he was being responsible and independent and then not reward that? Honestly, I put this trip out of my mind for a few years. It seemed too monumental to think about. Ultimately, we knew we had to figure it out.

I want to take you through the planning process here. This kind of stuff doesn't happen right away, and it doesn't happen at all, at least for us, without a lot of conversations and planning.

COVID canceled what would have been Benny's last year as a regular camper in the summer of 2020. We had barely thought about what it all might mean for the following summer when we got a notification that registration was open for Israel. This was in August 2020 and there was so much uncertainty! A generous donor wanted to do all they could to make sure the trip would happen. If we signed up early, we got a substantial financial discount. I held my breath and signed the forms.

That January, I reached out to the program to start having conversations. Turns out, they'd had a couple of T1D kids in this program before. Their feeling was that if we were willing to send him abroad at this age, he should be independent in his care, with the staff ready to act as a backup. Together, we decided we'd come up with our own plan and tell the program what we needed. They'd then let us know if they were comfortable with our requests.

I hung up the phone feeling a lot better about making it work. If they had asked if he needed to wear his pump the whole time or if their first question had been about liability, or a counselor losing sleep, I would have felt very different. But our expectations seemed to match. Remember, Benny had been at this camp for eight years already. While the staff in Israel wouldn't all be people he knew, we weren't talking to total strangers.

We then sat down with Benny and asked him what he thought would be a good plan. How did he want to manage? What were his expectations?

We talked about estimating carb counts and setting up several pump profiles to make it easier for him to adjust dosage. We do this for camp every year, with various profiles that decrease insulin across the board in different increments. Every pump brand currently in the US market has this feature, even if they call it different things. With Tandem, it's a matter of setting up different profiles. We'd used the Control-IQ AID system for a year and a half at this point, so we talked about using that system's Exercise mode, which targets a slightly higher glucose range.

We discussed the minimum number of blood sugar checks he'd do if something went wrong with the Dexcom. I called Tandem to order a backup pump for him to take along just in case; this is something most pump companies offer if you're out of the country or in a remote area for a long time. We talked about using long-acting if something really went wrong with the pump. And we talked about remote monitoring.

It surprised me to find that Benny wanted us to use the Dexcom Follow while he was overseas. We had agreed that we'd ask one counselor to Follow and that we'd set expectations for what the reaction would be if alarms went off. He thought it would also be helpful to have me as a backstop if his urgent low went off.

You may be nodding your head, saying, "Yes, that's a great idea." Most parents like the security of having Share and Follow when their child is away from home. Because I'm the Worst, I was not nodding. I was thinking, "What good is that? I'll be eight hours behind, and if your alarm is going off at 2:00 a.m., what am I supposed to do? Call the embassy?"

It was important to him, so we talked it out. We agreed that if his urgent low went off, I would wait at least fifteen minutes to text him. If he didn't answer and/or the urgent low went off for another fifteen minutes, I'd text or use WhatsApp to ping the counselor we'd selected. If I couldn't get a hold of the counselor, I'd go up the chain to other staff. I had contact info for several people in Israel and for those in the home office in the US. If it were an emergency, there would be a way to reach someone.

We also decided that I'd contact Benny and/or staff if his blood sugar stayed too high for too long. I noted in writing that our endocrinologist and I would agree on what that number/length of time would be. A trip like this is not the time to worry about perfectly straight lines or 100 percent Time in Range. I didn't want a staff member telling us that if he went over 160, the day was ruined. "Our doctor says . . ." usually goes a long way for these types of guidelines.

I didn't feel the need to go through a lot of emergency glucagon explaining or training. That's something we've done every year at camp, but Benny has taken it over. As I said in the very first chapter, anytime he's in a hotel room for a sporting event or on a trip with a friend's family, he shows his roommate his glucagon and explains what to do. He always tells them to get an adult and call 911 if he won't wake up or won't treat.

On this trip, one of the camp staff on site with the kids is also a medic, so while we didn't know what Israeli 911 would be, we were assured the medic would know what to do.

The next question I get after "How could you let him go?" is, "How the heck did you pack?"

We've been fortunate to travel a lot as a family, but what do you take for a month abroad? I scoured diabetes travel blogs and listened back to a podcast episode I'd done with a T1D family who traveled the world for a year. I looked at various packing lists and created my own.

We packed 50 percent more of everything and twice as many Dexcom sensors. Benny was skeptical he'd need that much, but it seemed like a good cushion to me.

The program asked the kids to pack two bags: a backpack that could hold three days of clothes and toiletries, and a larger suitcase that would stay on the bus or in the hotel, whichever was home base for that part of this trip. We packed an additional medical bag that would stay at a stable room temperature.

Insulin was tricky. They assured me it could be refrigerated throughout the trip and that other kids had medication that also needed to stay cool. This has been the case with almost every camp and school overnight program I can remember for both of my kids. Adding insulin to the "medical fridge" was never an issue. But this was an entire month on the road.

As you likely know, insulin is labeled as fine at room temperature for twenty-eight days and good for a year in the fridge. A new study from Doctors Without Borders shows that, under real-life conditions, insulin can be safely stored up to 99°F for up to four weeks.[18] That was reassuring, but we knew Benny would be outside in temps above 100°F, and who knows how hot the inside of his backpack might get!

We sent 50 percent more insulin than we thought he'd need on the trip and assumed it would stay refrigerated, but I was also prepared to toss anything unused when he got home. This was a difficult decision, because insulin is so costly and we hate to waste a drop. Ultimately, I had to do what was right for my son.

If you haven't thought about this before, it's easy to figure out how much insulin you'll need on a trip. Pumps will display the total daily dose (TDD) somewhere, although you may have to click around. We take the average of the last seven days (some prefer fourteen days) to find the average TDD. Multiply that by the number of days on your trip. Then divide by 1000 if you use vials or 300 if you use pens. You'll have to do the average TDD math manually if you're on multiple daily injections (MDI). Either way, that's a starting point. As I said, we sent 50 percent more.

We decided he'd always have an extra insulin pen in his backpack just in case. We tried a newer product, called VIVI Cap. I received this product as a free sample. It's very simple: you activate the cap and then you slide it onto an insulin pen instead of the regular pen cap. It keeps the insulin at room temperature. More on that in the next chapter; it worked incredibly well.

This system worked great. Benny carried what he needed in the backpack and every three days, he changed out his supplies. I was worried about charging the pump and his phone, but the program staff laughed. "These are all teenagers," they said. "They charge their phones and devices every day." That was true. We sent Benny with a powerful solar portable charger, but he said, except for the few days they camped in the desert, they almost always found a charging station wherever they went.

Benny has almost always used a camelback-type backpack, which means it holds a pouch of water. It's been fantastic for regular camp, and it worked just as well here.

One little ace up my sleeve; I knew that if Benny ran low on supplies, I'd be able to find someone in Israel who could help. Over my years of podcasting, I've made contacts all over the world, and I'd even had two advertisers based in Israel. But I didn't want to rely on their kindness, and I wouldn't have been able to do that in most other countries. Still, it made me feel a little reassured.

If you've ever sent your child to any kind of camp, you know there are a ton of forms. Imagine how many forms there were for this program! Now add on all the COVID forms we had to show in the summer of 2021. Israel was one of the most COVID-cautious nations, so it was a lot.

Once everything was packed and all the forms were filled out, we had one more big step: actually getting him there! The camp group would fly together overseas from Newark Airport, near New York City. The families were responsible for getting the kids to Newark.

My children are experienced flyers, but at this point, Benny hadn't flown by himself. My daughter had done two "unaccompanied minor" flights where you can bring the kids to the gate and then the attendants monitor them. Lea hated those, by the way. She had been fourteen and more than capable of managing herself, but under airline regulations, she not only had to be supervised (which I liked) but had to wear a giant 8.5" x 11" form in a lanyard around her neck (which I agreed was embarrassing). Benny was sixteen and, according to the airline, he didn't need the extra help at the airport.

I, on the other hand, worried he might need all the extra help he could get. Would he put his passport in his pocket, and have it fall out somewhere? Would he lose his phone? What if the plane was delayed? I wasn't too worried about any kind of diabetes emergency, but I was concerned that T1D could slow him down or make for an arduous trip.

I was also worried about the hassle of taking an entire month's worth of diabetes supplies through the domestic airport security. I couldn't imagine they see that very often! Benny had printouts of the program itinerary and documentation, just in case. I knew the Israeli airport security sees camp groups all the time, so they wouldn't bat an eye at this kind of packing. Of course, by then, he'd be with the actual group, along with staff that spoke Hebrew and was prepared to explain any diabetes airport issues.

We talked through a lot of my concerns and Benny shared a few of his own. We had one last great conversation about this terrifying and exciting trip and then he and my husband left for the airport. I'm embarrassed to admit that I didn't go. I was so nervous! I thought it would be better for him if I said my goodbyes at home. The last thing he needed was me crying all over him at the airport! I gave him giant hugs and tried not to throw up as soon as he walked out the door.

Benny had no issues going through security and getting to his plane in Charlotte. Easy flight to Newark and he met his camp group at their gate. That's when I started feeling a little better. The trip hadn't really begun, but he was with people who cared about him and would look out for him. He was so happy to be with friends and to take what he knew was a once-in-a-lifetime kind of trip. I was already proud of him.

I was proud of myself too.

ASK YOUR DOCTOR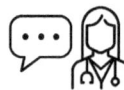

- Do you think my child is ready to travel independently with a non-diabetes group?

- Do you have any recommendations for packing or taking supplies on a long or international trip?

- If I ran out of supplies far from home, could your office help me get what I need? How would that work?

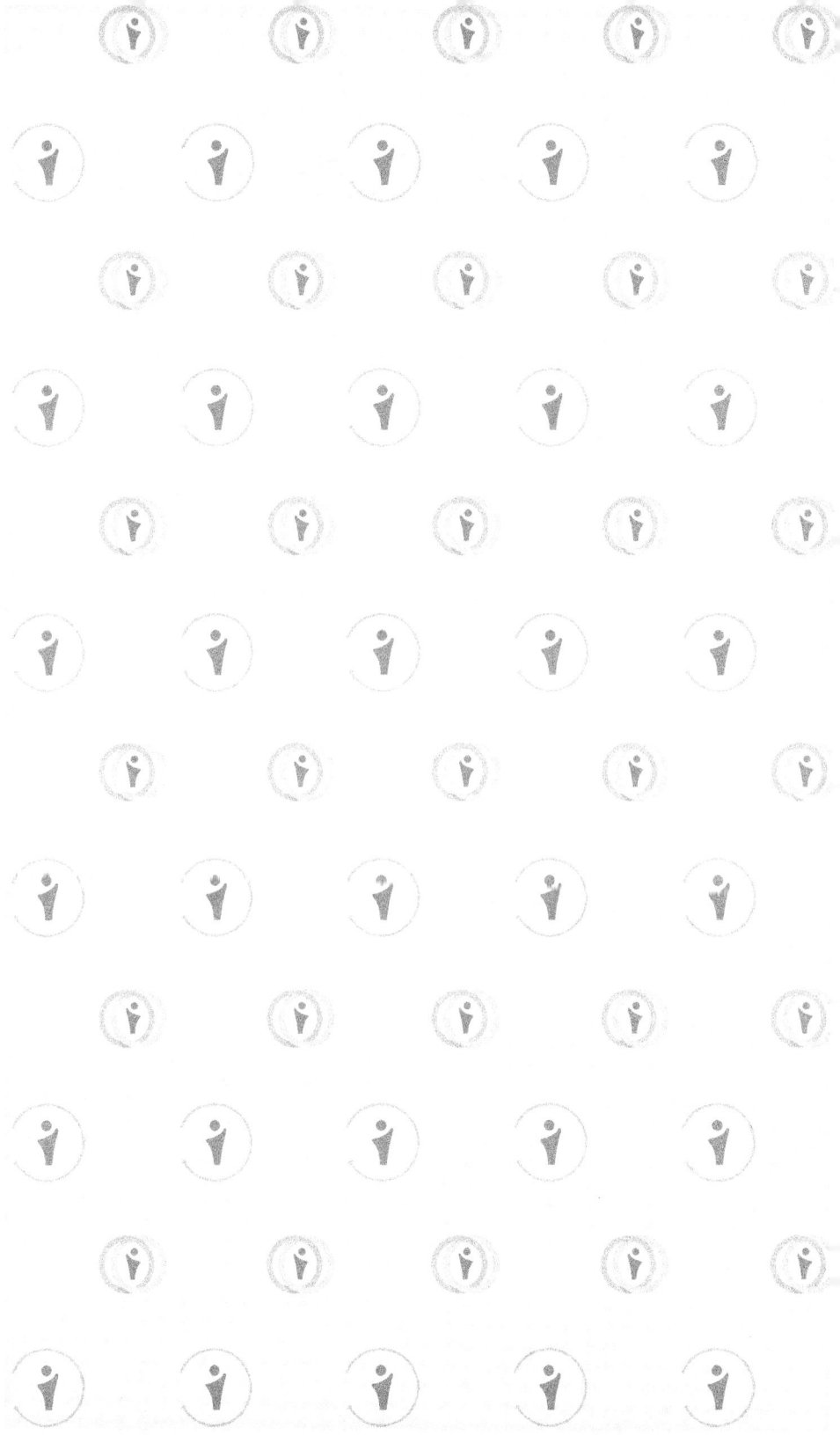

"There's no point in worrying about being perfect all the time. Because it's unrealistic. And it's not fun."

—Benny

CHAPTER 14

The Trip to Israel—the Reality

There's an old military saying: "No plan survives first contact with the enemy." For diabetes, that might be, "No plan survives first contact with real life!"

After committing to the trip to Israel almost a year prior and planning for over six months, the trip was underway! Let's talk about what happened, how we reacted, and what we'd do differently next time. I'll start by saying the trip was a home run. There were no diabetes emergencies. Benny took care of what he needed to and stayed in a safe range, and he had an incredible time. I also made it through!

Once Benny was home for a few days, we thought it would be fun to do a sort of debriefing interview on the podcast. I talked to him about the trip and asked some questions from listeners. I'm going to include quotes from that interview in this chapter, along with some of our texts and messages.

Once the group landed in Israel, the first order of business was SIM cards. For ease of communication and for security, they wanted the kids all on the same system. That meant changing out the cards pretty much as soon as they landed. Share and Follow still worked, and we realized we could communicate most easily through text when there was Wi-Fi and WhatsApp when there was not.

The kids had to quarantine for twenty-four hours before they started the actual trip and take one more COVID test. Then they were off! Benny switched to a much lower basal rate profile about three days into the trip as soon as all the hiking and activity geared up.

> **Benny:** About 20 minutes into the first hike. I immediately went low. The medic that was with us was great. She had prepared and had four hand-sized squeeze bottles of honey, and I downed like half of one, like 20 minutes into the trip. Battling those lows were ... the most difficult thing I had with diabetes pretty much the entire trip.

I asked whether the medic gave him a hard time or if he felt weird about asking her for help.

> **Benny:** No, she was cool. She was a medic in the Israel Defense Forces (IDF). She had worked with kids with diabetes before and she was fine about it. Eventually we got to the point where I just tapped her on the shoulder and she'd be like, "okay."

Because I know Benny will speak up, I wasn't really that worried about him getting help for low blood sugar situations. What I worry most about is diabetes stealing the fun and joy out of situations. I imagine everyone is engaged in an exciting activity and Benny must sit and wait for his blood sugar to go up. Or that other kids get nervous or think diabetes is weird and don't want to be around him. Luckily, he doesn't seem to worry about that very much.

Benny: I don't hang around people that would dislike me for something I can't control. I don't interact with those kinds of people. We almost never had to stop for me, but we stopped a lot anyway, just because everyone got tired. If we stopped because of me, everyone would be like, "Oh great, we're stopping. Thank you, Benny!"

Another of my fears is that diabetes will be front and center during these experiences, not the experiences themselves. Would he be looking at his Dexcom and worrying about a future low when everyone else was looking at a fascinating dig site? I asked him how often he thought about diabetes on the trip.

Benny: I wait until I get an alarm. It is not on my mind until something is wrong. I think it about it when I eat and I bolus but other than that, 90 percent of the time it's not on my mind, just in the background.

Sometimes I feel like diabetes is more in the background for Benny than it is for me. In a situation like this, I knew I'd have to actively work on a way to make sure I wasn't obsessed with the trip every minute of the month he was gone.

Having the numbers accessible made it harder for me. The temptation to stare at it all day and worry was very strong. I've mentioned before that when Benny goes to his regular non-diabetes summer camp, we don't remote monitor. Believe it or not, it's easier for me to not see those numbers. I know he's safe. They will call if there are any issues. I still worry, but after the first few days, it's easier.

For this trip, I talked things over with my therapist. I needed a way to check in without overdoing it and finding reasons to worry when I didn't need to. We decided that, assuming there were no urgent low alarms, I'd only look at the Dexcom numbers twice a day. I'd look when I woke up, which was afternoon his time, and I'd look again around 10:00 p.m.

Why those times? Of course, I had to look first thing in the morning! There is no way I could pretend I wouldn't wake up and grab my phone. So instead of fighting that, I made it official. I picked 10:00 p.m. because Israel is seven hours ahead of us and when it's 5:00 a.m. over there, that's close enough to his wake-up time that I could check to see if his overnight had gone well. It was also early enough in my evening that if there was a problem, I wouldn't be up super late trying to fix it. I'm proud to say I stuck to that plan; it worked very well for me.

What about food? Benny said that part was easier than he expected because they ate a lot of the same kinds of meals. Plus, he was exercising a ton and eating on a schedule, which always makes things easier. Diabetes loves a routine! There is no doubt in my mind that Control-IQ also helped quite a bit here. Under- or over-bolusing for food is less of an issue when you have a pump system helping you out.

One reason I'm comfortable sending Benny pretty much anywhere is because I know he'll explain the use of emergency glucagon to his roommates and counselors/staff. Knock on wood. We've never had to administer it in all these years. Now that there are easier options than just the scary "red box" options, I feel even better about it.

If you're not familiar, most doctors will say that everyone who uses insulin should have access to emergency glucagon. Glucagon triggers the liver to release its stores of glucose into the body, which raises blood sugar. Until just a few years ago, glucagon came in a red or orange box, depending on brand, and needed to be carefully mixed then injected with a very large needle. It was complicated and scary.

Since 2019, the FDA has approved three different, more shelf-stable versions of emergency glucagon. Baqsimi is a nasal spray; Gvoke and Zegalogue are two pre-mixed liquids that come in auto-injector pens or pre-filled syringes. We have prescriptions for Baqsimi and Gvoke, so I sent one of each with Benny.

The first day in Israel, Benny had a quick huddle with the three staff members who'd be with his group for the duration of the trip. He showed them the glucagon he'd brought along and explained how to use each one. Benny always tells roommates about using glucagon as well. On this trip, they'd switch roommates every time they were in a new city or town.

> **Benny:** Every night on the first night, I'd tell them how to use it. And I'd tell them NOT to use it unless they really couldn't get ahold of (the staff). "If anything happens, call Yoni (the head counselor). If you can't get ahold of Yoni, keep going up the chain until you get someone."
>
> **Stacey:** How did they react? Did anybody seem nervous?
>
> **Benny:** No. Everyone's super chill.

Luckily, no one ever had to break out the glucagon. I was shocked at how few urgent lows Benny had overnight. I give Control-IQ a lot of credit, along with Benny's hard work to treat before things got too low. There were a couple of false lows here and there. But nothing prolonged. His counselor, Yoni, was amazing.

> **Benny:** He'd text me in the middle of the night, you know, like 1:00 or 2:00 a.m. And he'd be like, "Do you need help?" because he'd wake up to the alarm. I'd tell him I was fine. And then in the morning, I'd go up and hug him and say I'm sorry for waking him up.

Yoni reassured Benny there was no need to apologize. He was there to help any teenager on the trip with overnight issues.

What about supplies? That plan worked out well too. Benny left his main medical bag at the hotel and took the three days of supplies in his backpack. He didn't use many extra pump infusion sets or Dexcom sensors. I think he was a bit more careful than he would have been at home and I know he used the overpatches on the Dexcom sensors.

I was appalled at the condition of his supplies when he came home. My neatly packed Ziplocs were gone, and it looked like he'd used his diabetes bag as a medical garbage bag too. But at least he wasn't trailing trash through the desert.

I had mentioned that we were trying out the VIVI Cap on this trip. That's a thermal insulin pen carrying case. You take the actual cap off your insulin pen and slide the VIVI Cap on; it looks like a bigger, beefier pen cap. The company is a bit cryptic about how it works, but it's insulated and absorbs heat and releases it back out into the environment. You don't have to charge it and it doesn't require water or ice. VIVI Cap doesn't keep insulin cold, but it keeps it at room temperature.

Benny usually uses vials, but just in case something happened with his pump, we sent a couple of pens. That way, he could easily switch to shots as a backup. He'd keep the VIVI Cap pen with him in the backpack and the other two pens would stay in the medical bag.

The VIVI Cap worked great! It's funny, Benny forgot all about it. He never actually used the insulin pen in his backpack. When he came home, he told me he didn't even remember it was there. So how do I know it worked? We did a bit of a test.

You're not supposed to use insulin that's been out of the fridge after about four weeks. Insulin is labeled to be stored at room temperature, below 77°F. This was a pen that had been out of the fridge for five weeks and had been in temperatures well above that, and probably above 100°F for sustained periods of time. Knowing all of that, and curious about the VIVI Cap, we pulled the insulin out of that pen and put it in his pump.

Amazingly, it worked just fine. We watched him carefully, of course, but numbers were in range. In fact, they were on the lower end of his range, probably because we were all watching so carefully! So big thumbs up on the VIVI Cap.

I think the only time I reached out to Benny unprompted about diabetes was the day before they were going into the Dead Sea. We'd been fortunate enough to travel to Israel as a family a few years earlier and we'd been very careful about that swim. They warn you about the salt content stinging your eyes or your skin, but we were most concerned about the Dexcom transmitter. For our family trip, we covered it with a big waterproof Band-Aid and I wanted to make sure Benny remembered to do that. I could see his eyes rolling as he texted back that he was all set!

Of course, he had a non-diabetes-related mishap. Benny is the kind of kid who finds a way to get a minor injury on every vacation. While they were snorkeling, he kicked a poisonous coral, hurt his foot, and had to go see a local doctor. It wasn't serious. They gave him some antibiotics and sent him on his way. Of course, they made sure Benny told us what had happened, but it was all cleared up in a few days.

One of my listeners asked Benny what advice he'd have for other kids who wanted to go away on programs or trips like this. Not necessarily a month abroad, but maybe to soccer camp for the first time or even an overnight school field trip without their parents.

Benny: It's going to be fine. If you know what you're doing at home, you know what you're doing anywhere. It might not be a month-long trip in a foreign country, it might be at your friend's house for a couple of days. But if you trust yourself enough to be able to take care of yourself for a couple of days, I think you should go for it. You're always going to have someone with you, or at least you should, that cares about you, and will do things that you need for you.

Stacey: You mean as a minor there is always an adult on these programs?

Benny: Yeah, there's always going to be at least two or three people that can and will help you with whatever you need.

This is what I mean when I talk about "not perfect, but safe and happy." You don't need all caregivers to be diabetes experts, especially as children with type 1 get older. You do need people who care and pay attention. It's also helpful that I have a child who's pretty easygoing about diabetes.

Benny: I mean, my thing is, you got to enjoy life. You can't worry about every little thing all the time. You know, you might live a full life and have perfect numbers. If you do good for you. You're the top 0.1% of diabetics. But there's no point in worrying about being perfect all the time. Because it's unrealistic. And it's not fun.

When Benny was heading home, this time I went to the airport. He came off the plane exhausted and hungry. He let me hug him for an embarrassing amount of time. It was fantastic!

ASK YOUR DOCTOR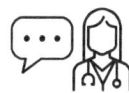

■ Do you have any recommendations to store insulin in extremely hot or cold weather?

■ Have any of your teen patients gone on adventures or international programs? What's worked for them?

■ Do you have recommendations for adjusting insulin dosing for this kind of travel or even for a more active vacation?

“ It was definitely 'our' condition for the first several years. However, being the parent of a child with diabetes is not at all the same experience of having diabetes. As Benny grows older, it's our job to do less and less. ”

CHAPTER 15

Customer Support

B enny's trip to Israel felt like a line in the sand when it came to his diabetes independence. We'd sent him halfway around the world and he'd done what he needed to do to stay safe and happy. Just after that trip, in August, we had our annual chat about the diabetes plan for school. How did he want to manage? As a junior in high school, what did he want from me?

"Customer support," he said.

I didn't understand. "What does that mean?" I asked.

"You know, customer support," Benny said. "I'll call you if I need you, but you're not asking me what's up." he explained.

That sounded terrible! Not because I thought he couldn't manage, but because it represented an enormous change from what had come before. How could the little boy who ran away from shots and insulin pump infusion set changes now be willingly responsible for all of his own care?

I agreed to try it if he kept his numbers within a safe range. We talked to his endo and Dr. V agreed this would be a great time to hand over control. If something went wrong or if Benny wasn't ready, we'd know right away and could jump in to help. As you know, I don't share numbers, but I will tell you that Dr. V and Benny's idea of "safe" is not my idea of "awesome." Even so, it all made sense and I reluctantly agreed to hand over the reins.

There's a duality to being a parent of a child with diabetes. Especially if your child is diagnosed very young, the parent does much, if not all, of the care. It can almost feel like the parent has diabetes; it was definitely "our" condition for the first several years. However, being the parent of a child with diabetes is not at all the same experience of having diabetes. As Benny grows older, it's our job to do less and less. I knew this moment of independence was coming, but that doesn't mean it was easy.

For many years, I said that the hardest transition we had was sending Benny to kindergarten. He'd already had T1D for four years and had a marvelous experience at our day care/preschool. Even so, I was terrified to send him to elementary school, and I was on edge for at least the first month.

Later, I decided that middle school was our toughest time with type 1. Benny had what I've learned is a very typical experience. He had the brain fog and forgetfulness typical of all tweens (including my daughter who doesn't live with diabetes) as well as the amazing physical changes, insulin resistance, and blood sugar roller coasters that can come with puberty.

If you ask me now, I'd say we're in another tough time, but this one is more about me. It's about letting go. We're transitioning into a completely independent management style. Benny is a year away from college and many of the schools on his list are far from home. Ironically, as Benny is getting older and more independent, I think about it more as "our" diabetes than I have in years.

Here's an example, but I have to warn you, it doesn't make me look very good! I speak out a lot against the pressure for perfection in our community. You may not realize that I'm often still fighting against that pressure in my own brain! This is the story of one of those internal fights.

This was in late 2019, when we were using Basal-IQ with the untethered method. Benny was in range before bed, hovering around 125. For the last few weeks before this, he'd been dropping about 15 to 20 points overnight. Just a little drop and then steady. I thought 125 was a fine number to just leave alone.

Benny texted me—yes, this is how we communicate in my house—that he felt low. I glanced again at the Dexcom and *in my head* I said, "You're not low. You're 125. I don't want to treat that.

You're going to mess up our great trend. And you're just going to go high. You're going to mess up our great numbers."

That's what I was thinking. Here's what I said, "Really? Because Dexcom says 125. You feel low?" And he said, "I feel like I'm dropping. See now I'm 117."

Even without the Dexcom number moving down a smidge, I knew my hesitation was selfish and misguided. Alright, it was dumb. He's not foolproof, but Benny knows his body. He'd been living with diabetes for thirteen years at this point; he didn't catch every low blood sugar, but he certainly knew what being low feels like.

I felt ashamed of what I had just been thinking. "You're going to mess up *our* great numbers"? Sadly, I have to admit I thought that. It's *his* diabetes. It's not *mine*. It's not *ours*. And there is no "messing up."

Chastened, I texted Benny, "Okay, I trust you. Let me grab you a drink. Do you think you need more than that?"

"Nope, just a juice box should be fine," he replied.

I grabbed a little can of pineapple juice, and I poured about twelve to fifteen carbs over ice in a highball glass, because sometimes it's just got to be fun. Yes, I was making up for my guilt with the splashy cocktail presentation. He didn't know that, but he got a kick out of it. He drank the juice and went right to bed.

I turned out my light, but I assumed I would hear that Dexcom high alarm soon. After all, I still believed I had given him fifteen carbs he didn't need. Instead, I woke up with my regular morning alarm. The Dexcom showed he had stayed between 100 and 130 all night long. He had been feeling low and he needed that juice.

A few weeks later, I attended a JDRF conference. I found myself with three adults with type 1 and I told them this story. Their reactions were interesting. They didn't tell me I was a terrible person. I was not told I was a helicopter mom. They simply said, "That's got to be tough." And "That sounds hard." But all three said it was important to remember, now that Benny is older, that those are not my numbers and it's not my diabetes.

They encouraged me to keep having these conversations—even just with myself. They pointed out that even though I'm struggling with how I'm thinking about diabetes, Benny is doing what he needs to do to stay safe and happy. They also encouraged me to realize that the move to independence is gradual and can be full of missteps, even for the parent. How could I have forgotten that last bit?! It was reassuring and eye-opening to realize that these adults with type 1 had gone through the transitions my son and I were experiencing. They'd struggled with independence and responsibility on their journey out of the teen years too.

Let's back up and talk about these transitions. As I said, it doesn't happen all at once. We didn't go from counting every carb and doing every injection at two years of age to letting Benny be completely independent at age seventeen. It's a gradual, thoughtful, and sometimes emotional process.

For me, it was helpful to consider diabetes milestones sort of like all developmental milestones. These all seem to be a combination of when your child is ready, when societal forces push them to be ready, and when the parent is ready to let go.

When Benny was five, we decided it would be helpful for him to do more with his diabetes care to make kindergarten a bit easier. Our daughter went to the school, so we knew we'd have very helpful educators and staff, but no full-time school nurse. That summer at our request, the preschool staff transitioned from doing all of his care to watching him do his own blood sugar checks with a meter and pushing the buttons on his pump to dose insulin. He always had an adult watching him, and they stepped in whenever he needed help. When "real" school started that fall, he just needed an adult who cared and paid attention looking over his shoulder. It was an immense help and he felt terrific about how grown-up he was.

I always like to point out, though, that was only the routine for school. At home he'd still hold his hand out to me to poke a finger, and we used his pump and meter remote to dose for him. Benny was far from fully independent, which I think is appropriate for a five-year-old!

I remember reading a post on Facebook from a mom of a seven-year-old who was asking why her son couldn't keep up with diabetes tasks. Why couldn't he be more independent? I was surprised. Who expects a first or second grader to be diabetes-independent? I kept reading and it turns out she had received some advice about how kids who were pushed to be independent with diabetes—to think about it as "their disease"—did better long term. I don't believe that's true. I certainly couldn't find any documentation, but who can blame her for wanting the best for her son? She was relieved when a bunch of us commented that independence comes more slowly.

I remember being worried because Benny seemed to be a bit behind other kids with T1D. He didn't want to do his own pump set changes until he was well into middle school, and we did all the Dexcom sensor changes until he was thirteen. He could perform those tasks, and he did them anytime he was away from home, but if we were around, he relied on our help.

While I was worried about Benny leaning on us "too much" at the time, looking back, I believe that reliance was actually an enormous help to him. It balanced the burden of diabetes until he was ready to shoulder more himself. I think one key to his current independence is that we didn't push. We knew there'd come a time when he didn't want our help anymore. We taught him how to do it, supported him, and let him figure it out.

That's why I mentioned earlier that it's helpful to look at diabetes readiness in a way similar to other childhood milestones. Before you protest that T1D is completely different, hear me out. When a parent of an elementary school-aged child asks me how they can set their child up for diabetes success, I ask them, "When was the last time you washed your child's hair?"

My daughter has amazing long and curly hair. One of her friends in kindergarten called it "mermaid hair," if that helps you picture it. Gorgeous, but hard to take care of. We struggled so much, combing it out when she was little and styling it as she got older. One day when she was maybe eleven or twelve, I looked at her bouncy, tangle-free curls and realized I couldn't remember the last time she'd asked me for help.

I also like to joke to parents of younger children that one day, the only time they will see their kids' underwear is when they're doing laundry. Remember when you used to have to get your kids dressed every day? For some children, that goes on for what seems like forever—even into middle school. No judgment, there are a bunch of reasons for that. But in almost every situation, that kid is going to wake up one morning and decide their mom will never see them naked again.

That happened to us with diabetes. Gradually Benny just didn't want my help. Every summer, I expected Benny to come home from diabetes camp or regular sleepaway camp where he did everything himself and be ready to kick me out of his care. It was much more gradual, and each step of management happened on its own timeline.

He figured out how to give himself shots—something he'd been very frightened of—when he wanted to take a pump break. He was ten and I told him he could go back to MDI, no problem, but that I didn't think he wanted me following him to school and around the neighborhood to do all of his shots. Benny agreed. He summoned up his courage and gave himself a shot. The pump break only lasted about four days, but he's been able to give himself shots ever since.

Another big turning point came when technology got better. Dexcom's G6 was released when Benny was thirteen. It has a much simpler applicator than previous versions. Who remembers the frightening design of the G4 and G5? The applicator was large and scary-looking, and the application was awkward. The G6 is a simple push button. Benny was nervous about the first application but wanted to try it himself. It went so well that in over four years since, I've never changed his Dexcom sensor.

That step forward helped him feel better about pump infusion sets as well. He was already doing those at camp and anytime he was away from home. I can't pinpoint the exact day he started doing them completely on his own, but it was sometime around the age of thirteen or fourteen. One day during his freshman year of high school, I realized the only way I know he's changing gear is when I hear giant coughs from the kitchen and when I see the diabetes trash in the garbage.

Do you know about the cough trick? I read a study years ago that coughing during injections alleviated pain. The researchers didn't know exactly how, but the idea is that the nervous system gets a bit confused and concentrates on the cough and not the pain. It works amazingly well for Benny; he does it for every infusion set and Dexcom change. Be careful if someone else is handling the needle, though; the person coughing may move or jerk suddenly and create an issue.

I'll credit more technology for another change, this one on my end. Because Control-IQ has been so helpful, I receive fewer and fewer Dexcom alerts. We already had a system in place where I don't text or call him for every alert and alarm, and between CIQ and him being responsive, I rarely had to reach out. This was also during COVID, so he was in the house most of the time! In the fall of 2020, I turned off the Dexcom high alert. In the spring of 2021, I turned off the low alert. Since then, the only alarms I get are for urgent lows (55 or below).

Do I still check Dexcom a few times a day? Of course I do! But not having all the alarms on my end gives Benny a chance to take care of situations and learn to troubleshoot without me texting him. There are even days when I only check in the morning and just before bed.

The one thing I couldn't seem to give up was asking, "Did you bolus?" Unless I physically saw him take the pump out and give himself insulin, I was always asking. Even after we switched to "customer support," this went on for a few months. He was getting annoyed, and it wasn't helping.

In January 2022, I decided I had to stop. No more nagging. I wouldn't ask about bolusing. I didn't tell Benny I was making a change. I simply did it. I wish I could tell you things magically got better and he remembered to pre-bolus for every meal. He didn't. What did change, though, was the tension.

Recently, "customer support" has stepped up just a bit. As I'm writing this chapter, in May 2022, Benny is having an incredibly stressful time. Junior year finals, ACT prep, his part-time job, and even some travel shoved in has made it a bananas couple of weeks. He's asked me for help with diabetes tasks, like filling cartridges, and I've pushed a little to see if it's OK for me to also remind him to change infusions sets and maybe even remind him to bolus.

I keep telling myself, this is why we gave him independence while he's still home. He needs to figure out how to make diabetes missteps in a safe environment. And I need to let him.

ASK YOUR DOCTOR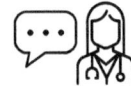

- Knowing my child's age and stage of diabetes, would you recommend any additional steps toward independence in care, either at school or at home?

- Can you share any technology tips to make insertion easier or recommend ways my child might help with management when they're ready?

- If my child is pushing for more independence, can you help us make a plan that keeps them safe and keeps me reassured?

" The fact that you were honest about diabetes attention definitely helped. If you had tried to lie about it or tried to hide it, it would have been even worse. **"**

—Lea

CHAPTER 16

Siblings—A Conversation with Lea

O ne topic I was eager to revisit this time around was diabetes and siblings. I don't know any parents in the diabetes community who feel they get this "right." T1D takes a lot of time and attention. There's really no way around that.

My daughter, Lea, is three years older than Benny. She was five when he was diagnosed. I thought it might be helpful to talk to her about this issue. What could we learn from a person who had dealt with a diabetes sibling almost her entire life?

What you're about to read is an excerpt of an interview that will air on the podcast shortly after this book comes out. I hope I don't have to say that we are a tight-knit family and the kids do really love each other. But we're also snarky and sarcastic, and I asked Lea to not hold back in this interview. She did not!

We don't have all the answers, but I think just having these conversations can be helpful. You may find your other children have surprising things to say about their perception of diabetes. They also will appreciate their feelings being validated and their voices heard.

Interview excerpt edited for clarity and to make it easier to read

Stacey: This is totally awkward. Hello Lea, and welcome to Diabetes Connections.
Lea: Hi mom (laughs).

S: You were five when Benny was diagnosed. Tell me a little bit about what, if anything, you remember about that time.
L: He had those sticky electrode things all over his body. And he was crying. He was very upset about it. I didn't really know what was happening. But I knew that my brother was crying and being annoying. It was really late at night and I'm like, why are we here? What's happening? This had never happened to me. I was like, "What's wrong with him?"

S: There were two days that you were with us. The first was the Monday we brought Benny in. When we thought something was going on. We went to the pediatrician's office. And for some reason, we all went. You came with us too. And we put you outside the room with your Leapster game.
L: Oh, the Leapster!

S: Because we didn't realize they were going to draw blood. He was screaming bloody murder because they had to do a blood draw. And we were like, "Don't worry, he's okay." And you were worried. Then, several days later, in the hospital, he was pulling those things off of his chest and we started calling him Baby Hulk.
L: Yeah, that's the memory I have of him.

S: One of the things that we purposefully did was, we decided not to ask you to be responsible for his diabetes. This didn't mean you didn't help. So fast forward to Benny going to kindergarten. And when he went to kindergarten, you were already in fourth grade.

L: The younger grades would sit towards the front of the bus, and the older grades towards the back of the bus. And it's a big privilege in fourth or fifth grade to sort of sit in the back of the bus. You're all cool. On the first day of fourth grade, rather than getting to sit in the back of the bus with all my friends, I had to sit in the front seat, right behind the bus driver, with my younger brother, because he has diabetes, and they want me to keep an eye on him. Now, up until this point, I have not been keeping an eye on this kid. This is not my problem. It was very quickly sorted out, but still some resentment there. I'm still mad about it, sorry.

S: Well, it's a very strange situation because we never asked for that. That did not come from us. We did give you both a talk about how you are responsible for each other. Not because of diabetes, but because you are brother and sister and you need to be there for each other. But as soon as we found out the bus driver had moved you, we fixed it.

You saw each other at school, but I don't remember a time where they ever called me and said you had alerted them to any issue with Benny.

L: The school is just big enough that you wouldn't see everybody all the time. But also, kindergarten and fourth grade are very different grades, very different situations. It was never something to worry about because to me, it was totally normal. Obviously, I understood that other people didn't have diabetes, but it was like, I don't know, my friend has this weird gray streak in her hair that's genetic. Everybody just has weird sh-t happening to them. You know? Can I curse on the show?

S: No, I'll take that out.

L: Tragic. But, you know, everybody has like weird stuff that they have or that they do. And it's just totally normal for them. Diabetes was just normal for me.

S: One of the things that I still feel bad about is how we handled bedtime a lot. Your father and I worked different shifts for a long time. Basically, he was the full-time morning parent, and I was the full-time evening parent. It was hard in some ways. (If I needed to do an inset change or other diabetes care at bedtime) I was giving you a book and saying, "Please read this. I know that your bedtime is after your brother's, but I've got to settle this crazy issue down."

I was exhausted. You know, I was getting up at 3:30 a.m. and by eight o'clock, I was a monster. And by nine o'clock I had no brain. That, to me, was one of the more difficult aspects of diabetes parenting because I tried to make bedtime a great time; you want to tell stories, you want to talk about your day, you know, and half the time I was like, "Hang on, hang on" And I'm sure you remember that.

L: It was never like you stuck me with a book I didn't want to read. I love reading. But when you would run to Benny's room, you would also leave his door open because you were trying to do both things at once. I could always hear you two talking. And I was just . . . jealous isn't the right word. But I was very aware of how much time you were spending with him at night. Because you never lied about it. I was very aware of how much time you spent with him. And what it was for.

You had to get the diabetes stuff done before bedtime. So that was the problem. It definitely stung a little bit. But it was also like I can just read the book by myself, I guess. Which is not a bad thing by itself, but I would prefer to have read it with you. But it's not something I can bring myself to be too upset about, even at that time. I knew you were going to be back, eventually. Then it'll be my turn.

S: I think even if Dad had been home every night, I don't think that you can give a child with diabetes and a child without diabetes the exact same amount of attention. It's just unfortunately, not how life works. And I think the way I managed it was to try to be honest about it, at least.

I think it's important to talk to your kids about it and to acknowledge that nobody likes diabetes. Yes, he gets more attention. It's not for the best reason, but that doesn't matter. Attention is attention. The other sibling is not going to say, "I understand perfectly now. Thank you for explaining." They're still going to be bummed. But in my opinion, honest communication, even with a five-year-old, at least lets them know that you respect them enough.

L: So that's definitely a big part of it is that if you're honest with your kids about what's happening. The respect is a big thing.

S: I did lie, though. I used to tell you everything I drank was coffee, because I knew you didn't like coffee. Because if I was having a Diet Coke or something I didn't want you to drink, I'd say, "It's coffee."

L: See, my mother is perfectly capable of lying to children (laughs). The fact that you were honest about diabetes helped. If you had tried to lie about it or tried to hide it, it would have been even worse because I was very aware that you and Dad were spending all this time with him. If you didn't give me this reason, maybe I'd think, "they like him better than me." Or "he's the better child." What is a child supposed to think? Even lies of omission and you're just not saying anything about it. That's almost worse, because, what are you hiding from me? Why won't you tell me? Is it something I did? Because there's no context from the other child, you're just spending all the time with them for seemingly no reason. So it must be something I did. But luckily, that did not happen.

And even in families without any chronic conditions, or anything like that, you know, you have a second child, and they obviously need more attention, because they're a baby and they can't do anything. And so it was already general sibling resentment of . . . Oh my God! I have to share everything now.

S: I think that's another difference between younger and older. I know a lot of families where the younger child does not have type 1 and they look up to their older sibling. They want to be supportive in a different way.

L: At one point, I was very intrigued by the meter. And so I did that once. It wasn't like, let me check my blood sugar all the time. Like, oh, I want to be like Benny. I want to check my blood sugar with him. But I don't want to get shots. I don't want to have to deal with counting calories, the *CalorieKing* book, how much food I'm eating, and then having to bolus for insulin.

S: It's funny, you said "calories" because of course, we don't count calories, we count carbs. But you mentioned the *CalorieKing* book.

L: Oh, the *CalorieKing*. And that's probably why I said calories. And you would go through and you'd find the foods that you were eating, and how many carbs were in them. That book was always at every meal. Somebody would have it. It would just be sitting on the edge of our table. I would just like read through it sometimes. It seemed like everyone was constantly looking at it. To me, it was cool information. But I didn't think, oh, I should start using it too. It was for diabetes. This is a diabetes thing, and therefore not my problem.

S: I'm glad to hear you say that, because one of the things we really were careful about was (restricting how our family ate). I wanted to focus on not creating an environment where disordered eating could blossom. I think we were very lucky. I mean, you have to be lucky, right? You, you could still do everything quote unquote, perfect. And you're still focusing on food so much that it certainly could have happened. But we also never said oh, that has this many carbs in it. You can't eat it.

L: No, you make a really good point about how it was never about too many calories or carbs. You also never used it as a cookbook. It was never like, oh, this has like fewer carbs. So we'll make this instead of that. It was always just oh, OK, you ate whatever you wanted. And this is how much you have to bolus for it. It was never, we're only going to bolus for this much so you can only eat this much and that's what we're going to make for you. And you never made different meals for Benny. It was never, "Oh, you're diabetic, so you can't eat that. We're going to make this thing for you. And we're all going to eat this food that you can't eat."

S: You may not remember this. When you were growing up, we had a rule that you had to tell us what you were eating. Now, that rule went out the window after elementary school, right? Because that was because you could reach the cabinets and you guys could both cook. I mean, you know, quote, unquote, cook. You could boil pasta. You could make eggs. You could make mac and cheese. You could make chicken nuggets.
L: Amazing. The core food groups.

S: But you could do that early on. I still remember when you and Benny started cutting things with knives because you know, Dad, he loves to cook. So we always had like these gigantic knives and he taught you guys how to use them. And I was like, oh my god, stop cutting fruit! Go eat some cheese doodles. (laughs) But my point was when you were younger, I used to say, let me know what you're eating. And that rule I made for both of you. Because I did think that would be a problem if only Benny had to say what he was eating. And literally it would be, "I'm eating goldfish." "Okay!"
L: I do remember yelling up and down the stairs, "I'm eating this!" It was very casual. But it's important that it was for both of us. It wasn't just for Benny because of his diabetes. And it wasn't just for me, because you thought I shouldn't eat something. You never said anything to me like, "A moment on the lips and forever on the hips." For me, you didn't say, "You shouldn't eat that much" or worried about weight or anything, which is so common for girls. You made it for both of us.

S: Alright, so let's talk a little bit more about diabetes and attention. Some of the things I tried were a little bit easier because we had a boy and a girl. So it could be you know, Dad's taking Benny somewhere and I'm going to take you on a girls' weekend, stuff like that. We tried to do things just the two of us, or even just with him, where you would get more attention and kind of be on your own. Did any of that sink in?

L: You know, there's general attention where it's like, you are a child, and you need love and attention to survive. And I got plenty of that. No worries. But it always felt like you had extra reserves of attention. And it was extra-credit attention, oh, if you want to do something fun, like, just the two of us, you know, if we want to do like a girls' trip, or if me and Dad wanted to go do something together, that always felt like extra-credit attention.

But it felt like Benny got all of the extra-credit attention all the time. And you know, whether or not that's true, that was my perception of what was happening. You know, a lot of this happened when we were very young. And I've, as I've already shown, I don't have very clear memories of it all.

There was never any solution that you offered, but there was never any solution you could have offered. There was there's no answer to this. And then you could never reassure me that it wasn't happening because it was happening. Which at the time just made everything worse, because I'm like, OK, cool. We're all acknowledging that this is happening. But there was nothing you could do about it.

S: That's hard for kids because you think your parents have the solutions.
L: Exactly.

S: I could have said, "Well, I will buy you a pony." But that's not the way we roll. It's hard. It's hard to sit here and listen to that because I want to fix it still. I want to go back and tell seven-year-old Lea, "It's okay." But I'm glad that I didn't lie to you.

Now you are in college finishing up your junior year. You're twenty. What's it like now? I mean, you're not around as much.

You're home for spring break now. But what is it like for you these days with diabetes?

L: When I first came home from college after, I think it was the winter break of my freshman year. First of all, he had a huge growth spurt. He became an entirely different person. Physically and mentally. He's like a real person. Now I can have a real conversation with him. He's still a seventeen-year-old boy, which is gross. But he has thoughts and feelings, which is a great improvement.

But the diabetes thing was still there. And so because I've never been able to disconnect the two of them, the diabetes was still there. Because yeah, I love him. But like, I have always resented part of him for it.

S: Do you worry about him at all? For diabetes?
L: Oh, absolutely not! No, but that's the thing. You never made it my responsibility. Sure, I understand the science behind it of what the pancreas is doing and how a pump works. But you never made it out to be this crazy, scary thing. Luckily, we've always had access to insulin. But it was never anything to be worried about.

Even if you had made it my responsibility as a child, I think I either would have ended up resenting you or just him more. Because, you know, if I had had to follow him because I was his diabetes protector, that would not have been great. Disruptions to social life are never great, especially if they come from a sibling, because it's like, 'Why do you get to live your life and I just have to follow you?' especially as an older sibling, because I was doing everything first. He got a phone before me because of his diabetes.

S: This again.
L: I got a phone when I graduated from elementary school, and I went to middle school. He got it while he was still in elementary school because of his diabetes. A lot of things that I was doing first, he would get earlier, which is a common thing with a lot of younger siblings anyway. But it was always with the caveat of: because of his diabetes.

I went to summer camp. And then he went to the same summer camp. And it was a whole thing because we had to go to camp early and talk to all the nurses and explain about diabetes. I was like, this is so stupid. This is my summer camp. I don't want to do this.

I've never been mad at him for having diabetes because that makes no sense. And he can't do anything about that. But, you know, I have no answer for how to get rid of it. I wish sometimes that I could get over that resentment sometimes.

S: Let's talk for a minute about social media. Because you're sort of my secret child. I don't post about you very often. I don't talk about you very often. And most of that is by request. Because years ago, you flat out asked me to not post much about you.

If you do see any posts with Lea on my Instagram or Facebook, she's approved it. Same with Benny. He adopted that after you. I think as a parent, it makes it a little harder, because I see lots of my friends posting a lot more. But I also feel good about it. I am curious. You're a kid with no social media. You had a little social media when you were a senior in high school. What's up with that? Do you remember what you were thinking and do you think it has benefited you in the long run?

L: So, moms can be embarrassing. Parents like to do lots of funny things with their young kids. They do all kinds of weird photo shoots or just funny family pictures or whatever. And that was all very embarrassing as a child. Especially because when I was in middle school, you know, peak cringe. I don't think it was ever like "to protect the privacy of your children, you should not post about us without our permission." It was more just I was an uncomfortable, gross tween. And I didn't want you posting pictures of me and my uncomfortable grossness.

But, you know, as I've grown up with the internet, there are a lot of people who do that. They post random pictures of their children without thinking about it. Especially very young children with things that other people should not be aware of.

But I'm really glad that you didn't. Because then I just don't have to worry about it.

S: I'm very proud of you. I joined Facebook and Twitter in 2008. So you were seven. And I was blogging a little bit before then. I could have done as many parents of children with diabetes and other chronic conditions have done—I could have put my children front and center. We could have named the blog after you and Benny. And I could have done that. But I thought at the time, it was not a good idea. And I still think it's not a good idea. Even having written an entire book about you and your brother's childhoods, we've left out a lot of personal stuff. I'm very careful about what I share publicly. And we talk about a lot of it before I do it. And I think it would have been a big mistake for our parenting and family style to be like "here's the Benny & Lea Blog!" I just I don't think that would have set you up for success.

All of that to say, I don't wish you were more part of my diabetes social media. I do think that what you're doing, even just with something like this, is really generous and will help people. I mean, of course, now I wish I could go back and redo parts of your childhood. But that's not how it works.

L: I mean, it turned out fine. It's not like you messed me up.

S: Did you . . . have you ever considered your career path? Have you ever considered advocacy or anything like that because of diabetes? Okay, you can be totally honest, because I think the answer is absolutely not.

L: The answer is absolutely not, but not for the reason you might think. It's not because of Benny. I just wasn't interested in it.

S: You're a geology anthropology double major, which is very cool.

L: Yes, very unrelated to diabetes.

S: Well, Lea, thank you very much for joining me. This has been really fun. Love you, sweetie.

L: Love you!

❝ Driving was not a rite of passage I was looking forward to. But as with every stage of parenting, you have to decide how to tackle it, how hard to manage it, and when to let go. **❞**

CHAPTER 17

Driving and Diabetes

T here are few things more exciting to most teenagers than getting their driver's license. There are few things more stressful for the parents. Add in diabetes and seeing your child get behind the wheel may be one of the biggest stressors we can face. It certainly has been for me.

I talk about learning from mistakes a lot, but this is one case where your mistake can hurt someone else. This chapter will probably be a bit more serious than the rest of the book, but that's on purpose. I had a scary brush with diabetes and driving years before my son's diagnosis and it's stayed with me.

Just after college, a friend with type 1 crashed his car on the way to work. He just passed out behind the wheel, I assume from a low blood sugar. Luckily, he wasn't badly hurt, but it was a serious wreck and the car looked awful. As you can imagine, almost thirty years ago, the technology was very different; my friend didn't have a pump or a CGM and he was using the older, less predictable insulins. Those differences have made things better, but of course, they haven't made things foolproof.

I've tried to make my friend's experience a cautionary tale for me and not a horror story. Like a lot of diabetes parents, I started thinking about driving long before giving my child the keys.

In our state, North Carolina, you can take a driver's education class as early as fourteen-and-a-half and get your permit at fifteen. That means you always have to drive with an adult in the car. A graduated license starts at sixteen—you can drive by yourself only between 5:00 a.m. and 9:00 p.m. Six months later, you are eligible for what the kids call their "after nines." At eighteen, you get a full license; no real change, but the license itself switches from vertical to horizontal layout to show you're no longer a minor.

In terms of diabetes rules and regulations, check with your state's Department of Motor Vehicles (DMV) and talk to other families who've been through the process. Many states have special licensing rules about medical conditions; almost all of them are different. I'll be honest, for us, in North Carolina, it was clear as mud. I'll explain.

Benny goes to public school, but my daughter attended a private high school and we really liked the efficiency and ease of the driver's ed course she took. It was a scheduling issue more than anything else; there was just more availability for our busy schedules, so we signed Benny up.

I informed the school that he had type 1 and wore a pump and CGM. We shared our agreed-upon strategy for checking blood glucose before driving (more on that soon). The organizer and instructors didn't bat an eye. Benny was far from the first child they had in this school with type 1. The owner sent me a link to the DMV forms about driving with diabetes.

I filled those out and had them signed by our endo, but no one officially ever asked for them. I even called the DMV and was told that if no one had specifically asked, then there was no case number and no one to send the forms to. They told me they would not accept them if I mailed them in without a case number; they'd end up in the trash. Really?

Meanwhile, our friend who went to a public-school driver's ed was pulled out of the class because he'd checked the box saying he had diabetes. He needed to submit those forms and he had to reschedule the class.

I run a large local Facebook group for parents of kids with type 1. We both posted about our experiences and found that—public or private—almost every teen had a different experience. It's so frustrating! Some parents recommended you just not disclose, but that doesn't sit right with me. I think it's important to disclose if asked. There are insurance and liability issues and we've spent these kids' childhoods telling them not to hide their diabetes. Why would we tell them to do the opposite now?

After a lot of conversation, we think the difference may have been the actual forms the kids received. Ours asked us to check a box if the person had ever had a medical event or took medication that led to a seizure, diabetic or otherwise. Other parents had a form that asked if they just had a medical condition, such as diabetes. I have no idea why there would be two forms, and in discussion with other parents, it didn't seem to matter if the driver's ed classes were public or private school; the forms varied regardless.

Moira McCarthy's excellent book, *Raising Teens with Diabetes*, addresses driving very well and she even has a contract for your teens to sign.[19] We did this with Benny. The technology has changed since she crafted that chapter, but the thinking is the same.

Moira (and almost every expert) recommends that people with diabetes know their blood glucose every time they get behind the wheel. It's easy to find out if your teen is doing a fingerstick—you can just look at the meter later. But how do you confirm a glance at a Dexcom graph on the teen's phone?

When Benny was learning to drive, we used the Road Ready app to keep track of driving hours. I'm sure there are others out there, but this was very easy. It emails info to the parents and gives you a simple printout of the log for the DMV. It also ensures your child is using their phone every time they get in the car but before they start driving. If they don't log those hours, they can't get their license.

We took advantage of that. After Benny finished with the Road Ready app, he was to open the Dexcom app and look at his number. We decided no driving below 90 or above 300 to start. That high is less about being impaired, at least for Benny, and more about just not feeling great behind the wheel.

This was easy when he had his permit because an adult was always in the car with him to make sure he checked. He got into the habit very quickly, but I didn't want to rely on his habit all the time. How to verify? I asked Benny to take a screenshot of his Dexcom every time he got behind the wheel. It was an extra second to add to the routine: Open Road Ready app, open Dexcom app, screenshot, done. He did that for the first month or two after he was allowed to drive on his own.

One of my proudest parenting moments was soon after Benny got his license. He was heading home from wrestling practice and texted that he would be a little late. He'd pulled over because his Dexcom had alerted he would soon be below 80. He was treating and would just wait it out.

It's hard to express how exciting it was to get that text. I was absolutely overjoyed! He told me where he was—in a church parking lot about ten minutes from our house. I was so pleased that he didn't decide to just tough it out and drive those last few minutes. Smart and responsible.

Of course, a few minutes later, I was back to freaking out. He asked if I could start heating up his dinner. I don't know about your kids, but high school schedules can be brutal, and during sports or theater activities, we rarely ate all together. Benny would often come home from wrestling at 7:00 or 8:00 p.m. and heat up whatever we'd left for him. I assumed this meant he was on his way; after all, it only takes a minute in the microwave.

But then ten minutes went by and he wasn't home. Fifteen minutes. Where was he? That parking lot is almost around the corner from us. Did he not come up from the low? Did he have a regular nondiabetic crash? I was really starting to panic when he texted, "Blood sugar is going back up. I'm on my way." He hadn't started driving after giving me the dinner order! Looking back at the texts, it was clear I had just misunderstood. Whew!

Truly, a really proud moment for me. No big deal for him. He was doing what we'd agreed on. But wow! I was so happy.

It was also great that he didn't freak out when he got the alert. He safely pulled over. That was something we'd talked about when he had his permit. I told him he needed to stay calm and not just stop in the middle of a busy highway or in the middle of the median if the Dexcom goes off.

An eye-rolling "really Mom?" moment, but I think it's important to talk about these things. These kids don't know what they don't know about driving. Moira was invaluable in reminding me to talk to both kids about where to safely pull over if needed—not just for low blood sugar—and where to park safely to wait things out.

In terms of treating, Benny has always relied on juice boxes and sometimes Gatorade or glucose gummies. He has always hated tabs. When we talked about what to leave in the car, I pictured always restocking Gatorade and, frankly, I worried about him getting the cap open. I've heard stories of adults with lows who struggled to open the juice bottle or stick the straw in a juice box!

"Mom, just give me a bottle of tabs," he said. And just like that, the kid who never wanted to eat a glucose tab—we're talking fourteen years here—saw that a bottle of tabs that won't freeze or melt was a lot more practical than his usual options. I think that's partly a sign of him growing up, and partly a sign of just how badly he wanted to drive! Either way, I'll take it.

If your kiddo really prefers something else, I've heard Skittles, jellybeans, or Starburst are great options. Again, you're looking for something that can't melt or freeze, depending on where you live, and sugar that's easy to open and consume if someone is by themselves.

When the kids were younger, I drove a minivan for probably about twelve years. I joked I could live out of that thing for a week—there were so many snacks and supplies in it. I don't think Benny wants to do the same in his car, but I think it's a good idea to have backup stuff. Not just diabetes stuff. You want a tire gauge, a flashlight, and a first aid kit, right? When I lived in upstate New York, I also had a blanket just in case, and I always like to have water in my car. So why not throw in a little backup diabetes kit with at least a meter, a protein bar, and a few emergency glucose tabs?

I think everyone with a medical condition should wear a medical alert bracelet or necklace. Some feel an ID medical card in the wallet is enough. Lots of adults with T1D get tattoos. Whatever you choose, I believe your child must wear something that identifies they have diabetes. To me, a seat belt cover or relying on their insulin pump isn't enough. In a severe accident, they may be thrown from the car or the pump may be ripped off. Again, scary stuff to think about but important to address.

If your teen has resisted a medical ID, driving may be a powerful enough motivating factor to get them to change their mind.

What happens if you find out your teen is driving low or otherwise breaking the rules of your diabetes contract? This is a tough one because getting a license is exciting! It means freedom—not just for your teen, but for you! You've probably got more time for yourself because you're not driving your kid everywhere anymore. But the stakes are just too high to let them break the rules.

It's hard to hear, but if they hurt someone, your child can face jail time. And, of course, they will have to bear the guilt and trauma that could go along with hurting someone else. Because of this, most experts recommend taking the keys away for the very first infraction; you can put that in your contract. Length of time is up to you, of course, but if it's painful—like two weeks or even a month—it's a good bet it won't happen again.

Driving was not a rite of passage I was looking forward to. I hated when both kids started driving. But it's part of our lives. Like everything with parenting, you have to decide how to tackle it, how hard to manage it, and when to let go.

Driving is also a time when parents who haven't yet turned on a tracking app start thinking about using one. This subject could be its own book, but let's touch on it briefly. There are a bunch of phone apps that make this easy and newer cars have a GPS built in. My advice here is that if you decide to turn on Life360 or Find My Friends for your child with diabetes, you need to turn it on for every child in the house.

Our rule has been that anytime our kids leave town or are on the road for more than an hour, they share their location via an app. My daughter will be twenty-one soon, and I'm going to ask that she continue to share for long road trips and unusual situations. But it will be her decision.

I think a helpful way of looking at these trackers is to not assign a value to them. There is nothing inherently good or bad about the apps themselves; it's about how you use them. I wouldn't want to track my kids (or my spouse or my parents) without thinking it through and having a conversation with them about it. First, what's the purpose? What are the parameters? And what's our agreement about communication and consequences?

It's ultimately a parent's decision, but this is a lot like the conversations around remote monitoring of a CGM. Let's say you have your child turn on the tracking app. Could you agree to not text your child if they're home on time, they check in with you regularly, and they aren't getting into trouble? But agree if that if they don't answer a text after a certain period of time or if you see their location is odd or looks dangerous, then you're going to act.

There's a good argument to be made about personal growth for the children here too. A lot of parenting experts will tell you that over-tracking children creates more fear in them and can reduce independence in the long run. You know my parenting philosophy is about learning through mistakes. I want my kids to learn the same way, within reason. It's a tough one for sure.

One last note here. We drive a lot and now that we have four licensed drivers, it actually makes those long car trips a little easier. Last year, Benny and I took a trip to Florida, just the two of us; Lea was still at her school and Benny wanted to visit friends from camp. The camp is in Georgia, but it seems like all of his friends live all over Florida! We split the driving on the way down. At this point, he'd been driving for two years and had his full license for one year. I will not lie—I was vigilant. No naps, and I had my eye on the speedometer the whole time.

On the way home, I loosened up. I felt more confident in his driving. I did close my eyes for a bit, but first I told Benny if he got a speeding ticket, he'd pay the fine and lose driving privileges for two weeks. It was I-95, so I wasn't worried about us being the fastest car on the road! I got my nap, and he did great.

Being alone in the car with him all that time gave me the chance to learn what music he's listening to these days and to have some great conversations. I never thought I would miss our back-and-forth driving all over town when he was in elementary and middle school.

Driving is a huge milestone for any teenager and their family. It's the end of an era and the beginning of something new. I don't think I'll ever really stop worrying, but that's nothing new. As always, I've got to give him the tools he needs to stay as safe as he can, and then let him hit the road.

ASK YOUR DOCTOR

- Can you help me figure out what our state requires for driving with diabetes?

- Do you have any concerns or advice about my child being safe behind the wheel?

- What range do you generally recommend for driving?

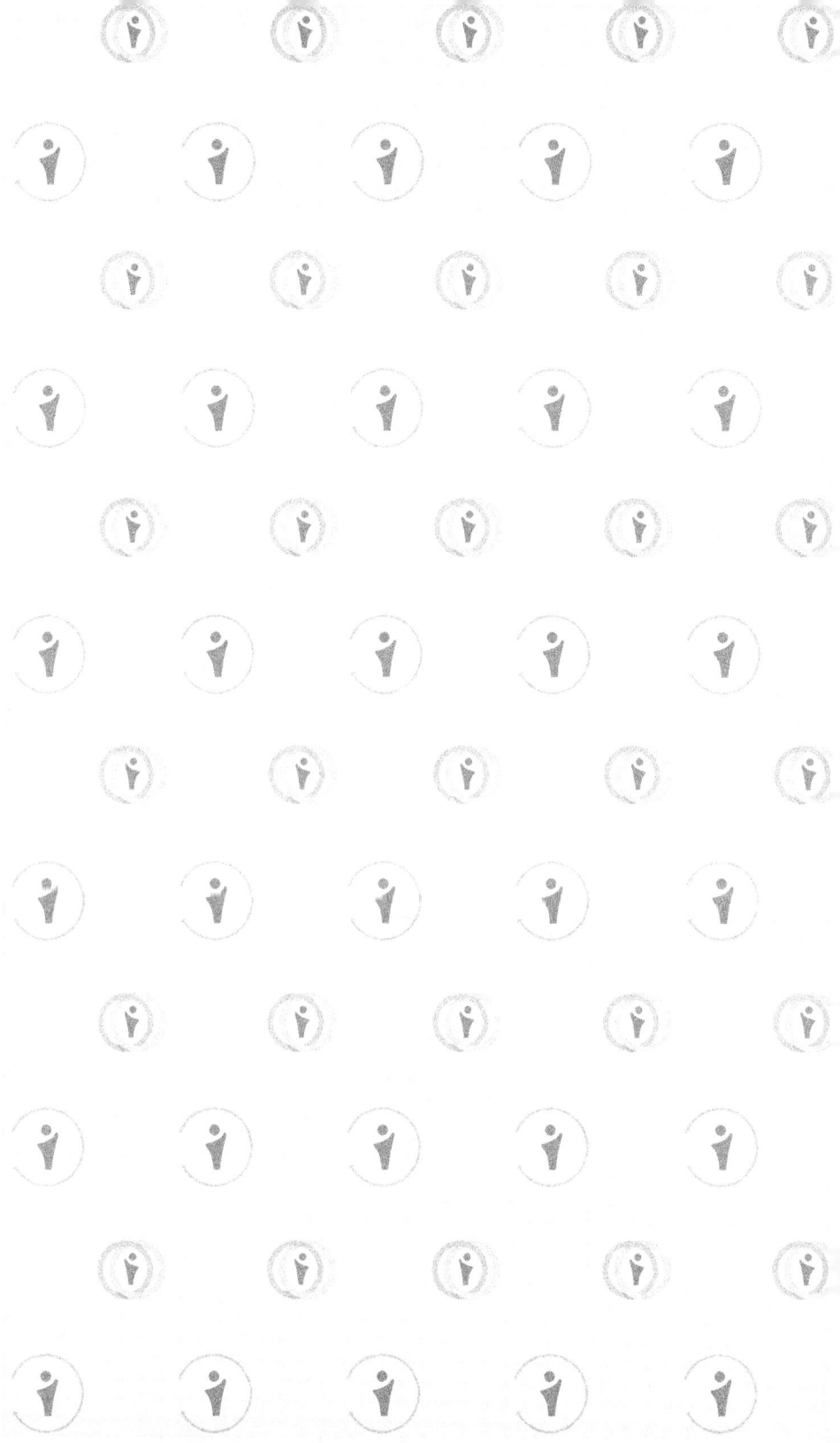

" These should be some of the most fun and most relaxing times with your family! Having to stress out about diabetes technology sticking when you just want to splash in the pool is no fun. "

CHAPTER 18

Get Your Gear to Stick

For many summers, I dreaded Wednesday nights. That was spaghetti night at our local pool. You could get dinner for the family at a cheap price and the kids could play, splash, and swim for a few hours. It was fantastic and fun until Benny would run by my chair yelling, "Mom, my inset came out!" Ugh! It happened quite often when Benny was little and we were new to pumping.

One of the hardest parts of using an insulin pump, for us, was keeping the infusion set stuck to Benny's body. It would come off in the bathtub or the pool, even on very sweaty days we had to worry about it sliding off! Finally, about two years in, I learned about sticky skin barrier wipes like Skin Tac. It made a tremendous difference to us!

When Benny started wearing a CGM, we quickly realized we needed extra help to keep that stuck to his skin, especially in the wet summer heat. Skin Tac was OK in winter, but we reinforced it with overlays when it got hot. It took us a long time to find something that worked well.

It's so frustrating because these should be some of the most fun and most relaxing times with your family, right? Just seeing the ocean water on a beach trip feels like it lowers my blood pressure. Having to stress out about diabetes technology sticking when you just want to splash in the pool is no fun.

Hopefully, our experiences can help keep your little ones' gear on even when it gets wet and wild! Here are some non-medical mom tips we've learned over our years on the beach and in the pool. Please note, because everyone's skin is different, this can take a lot of trial and error.

It's worth taking a few extra minutes to do a little prep before applying anything on the skin. If possible, the best time for a new infusion set, pod, or CGM is fresh out of the shower or bath. Make sure the skin is clean and dry; a few swipes with an alcohol pad can help too. You want to make sure the application area is free of moisture from sweat, lotion, or even natural skin oils.

Timing is important too. This is less about the time of day; I can't imagine anything sticks better in the morning compared to late at night. (But let me know if that's true!) What I'm talking about is time-to-water. Ideally, you'd let a pump set or a CGM sensor stay stuck for at least twelve hours before you jump in the pool. Real life dictates that's not always possible, but try to leave yourself at least three hours before getting the site wet.

I highly recommend using a sticky skin barrier. Products like Skin Tac and I.V. Prep do double work here. They help provide a thin extra layer to protect most skin from irritation and they make the skin tacky. For us, this is all we need almost anytime to keep technology stuck tight. Some people also apply it on top of the sensor/infusion set tape, but we don't find that to be necessary.

Skin Tac comes in a bottle and in wipes. We prefer the latter; if you use the bottle, be *very* careful not to spill any of it! This stuff is made to be very sticky and if you spill it, you're going to have to do some serious cleanup (keep reading for the "remover" version). These days, Benny doesn't even touch the actual wipe. He rips the package and nudges part of the wipe out of the top. Then he holds the bottom of the packaging to apply the exposed part of the wipe to his skin.

Many people will paint a "donut" or O shape on the skin to leave the area where the sensor goes into the skin free from the liquid. We had never been advised to do this, so we never did. Hasn't made a difference. We are extremely lucky with infusion sets and sensors and get the full length of use out of, I'd say, 90 percent of them.

Insertion technique is important as well. Every brand is a little different, but most recommend you run your finger over the tape surrounding the sensor or infusion set, wherever the sticky part surrounds the cannula or the wire meets the skin. Read the directions or watch the company's video. Securing that sticky tape by pushing down lightly around it a few times can make a big difference for some people.

As I said, it may take trial and error to find what works. We have had no luck with I.V. Prep, but my friend swears by it for her child. The only brand of overlay that works consistently in the toughest conditions, such as ocean and camp, for us, is StayPut Medical, but our T1D babysitter loved GrifGrips. If you haven't found what works, keep trying. Ask friends (and the companies) for samples!

Other popular brands include Opsite Flexifix, IV3000, Tegaderm, Pump Peelz, ExpressionMed, and RockaDex. Dexcom has its own brand of overlay and will send it to customers for free. You can find more overlays and bands at sites like www.uselesspancreas.com.

Years ago, Benny was at summer camp while I attended a conference. I was having dinner with the wonderful diabetes writer, Kerri Sparling, when I got a call from the camp nurse. Benny was with her and they wanted me to know that in the first week of camp, he'd already gone through three sensors. Something had knocked the first one off and the other two slid off because of sweat.

I asked to put Benny on speakerphone. Since Kerri knows more about diabetes than I ever will, we asked what she thought. Kerri asked, "Would it help to shave where you put the sensor?"

Benny laughed. "What? I'm not that hairy!"

Not a bad suggestion, though. We talked through moving the Dexcom off his preferred area of the arm and to his stomach, just for camp. That might protect it better. And there's less hair. I promised to ask around at the conference as well. The next day, I met the guys from StayPut Medical. They make overpatches for just about every type of diabetes technology. Mike gave me samples for Benny. We sent them to camp and, amazingly, our troubles were over. It's the best overlay we've ever used.

If your skin is easily irritated or you want something you can take on and off, a sleeve or a band may do the trick. You're limited to arm placement here, but Dexcom is approved for use on the arm in Canada and the UK. As far as I know, American arms are pretty much the same! Seriously, I'm told when Dexcom G7 approval comes in the US, it will include "alternate sites" like arms. So you won't have to feel like you're breaking the rules anymore.

A very popular and inexpensive option is vet wrap. Vet wrap is a self-adhering bandage, so it sticks to itself but not to other surfaces. It's used a lot for horses and other animals because it doesn't stick to hair or fur. Comes in very handy for people too!

Fun fact: vet wrap is actually called a cohesive bandage, but the brand Vetrap (that's how it's spelled) has become synonymous with it. Sort of like Kleenex or Xerox. So when people talk about it, they usually just use the common spelling "Vet Wrap." Either way, this never worked for us. I either never learned to wrap it correctly or we didn't wait long enough before going into the water. So I can't recommend this one, but a quick Facebook search will show that we are in the vast minority; most people love it. You can find lots of colorful types of vet wraps on Amazon or in animal supply stores.

We never used a sleeve or band. While I thought they were a great idea, Benny never wanted to try any of them. I have ordered and returned quite a few over the years! They all seem like they'd work well. It was more of an aesthetic thing for him—he just didn't like the look. In my opinion, SleekSleeves makes beautiful device covers. Deck My Diabetes and Bands for Diabetics are also good go-tos. I know parents who've cut up athletic shirts or repurposed wrist sweatbands. Have I mentioned we're a creative bunch?

For a more basic solution, we have slapped a giant waterproof bandage over Dexcom sensors and pump infusion sets. This is great in a pinch when you run out of supplies, or when you need to protect the transmitter. Most of the patches I mentioned earlier have a cutout for the infusion set or CGM transmitter, but there was one time we wanted it covered.

We swam in the Dead Sea a few years ago. It has incredibly high salt content; there are warnings all over the place about how any cut you have on your body is going to sting and you never want to put your face in the water. They also warn about taking any medical equipment in with you. I wondered, Could the high salt content damage the Dexcom transmitter? We decided not to risk it. Benny applied a large Tegaderm clear waterproof bandage over the top. He peeled it off a few days later—while the sensor was still on—and it worked out fine.

The best part about using a waterproof bandage is the convenience. You can buy many brands at your local pharmacy—no special order needed. How often do we get to say that with diabetes stuff?

Some insurance companies cover the cost of some of these products, so be sure to ask.

With over sixteen years in the diabetes community, we've heard a lot of interesting techniques. I know someone who uses a hair dryer to "set" the overlay she uses. That didn't work very well for us, but she swears by it. In a pinch, you may have seen photos of duct tape and other household fixes. That's probably going to irritate some skin, but with the cost of medical supplies—and the inconvenience of calling them in—it's no surprise people get creative!

What about removal of this very sticky stuff? I don't recommend Benny's method, which is to just rip it off. There are gentler methods, especially for younger children and anyone with sensitive skin. I recommend StayPut Medical's Release—Adhesive Remover, but there are lots of brands such as Uni-Solve and TacAway. Even baby or coconut oil will do the job.

Once you find what works, it goes a long way to relieving the stress of swimming and sweat. I have to warn you, though, Benny has had some ridiculous tan lines. When he was younger, he saw that big Dexcom patch oval as a sort of badge of honor. But as he got older, he thought about placement a bit more. Just one more thing to think about with diabetes, right? To that end, be very careful about sunscreen near these patches or any diabetes devices. Omnipod, especially, can be sensitive to sprays (they can cause cracks in the Pod's casings), but lotions and even bug spray can be an issue. It's a good idea to apply sunscreen with your hands around the sites.

Benny's biggest tan line came after an epic summer Dexcom run. In 2019, he put on a sensor just before diabetes camp and secured it with a large blue StayPut overlay. The sensor stuck perfectly during the entire week of camp, including water play, swimming, and sweat. A few days after he came home, we took off for a couple of days at the beach. The sensor was set to expire, but it was sticking so well we restarted it.

There are a few DIY ways to restart a Dexcom sensor. That's not at all medically recommended, so I'm going to play it safe and ask you to google it (there are a bunch of videos on YouTube to help). That sensor stayed stuck tight to Benny's arm for a full two weeks. We'd brought along Jackson, Benny's best friend, to the beach and they played in the waves and in the sand for three days. That sensor, and that overlay, were amazing!

I took Benny and Jackson to the beach while my husband took our daughter to an admitted student weekend at her college. Benny and I love the beach and Slade and Lea aren't as big fans, so it worked out great. I set out some rules for the boys—basically the big one was no swimming in the ocean unless I was physically on the beach at the time.

I had a lovely spot—chair and umbrella, a book, and a bunch of podcasts. During this trip, I was actually working on the cover and edits for book one! But what I really remember was monitoring the boys, not just for safety, but to see if the Dexcom was staying on! I was using my phone to zoom in as close as I could on his arm. It was the most amazing sensor run I think we ever had!

The last big challenge we've had for keeping diabetes tech stuck to Benny's skin was when he wrestled. This was the first two years of high school. After a lot of trial and error, we found that athletic tape worked well around the Dexcom. He had the athletic trainer tape it "super-secure" for meets. The pump infusion set stayed on easily for meets (he removed his pump). For long and sweaty practices, he found that taping it with Opsite Flexifix or another full overlay worked best. He wouldn't even cut a hole for the tubing; he'd just slap the tape over the entire thing and then gently remove it after practice. Not my ideal, but it worked for him.

When I talk to the folks at Dexcom for the podcast, they say the upcoming G7 will have a new adhesive. This is supposed to be just as sticky but less irritating for most people. I'm excited to see how it works!

We've learned a lot since the days of Wednesday spaghetti night. Diabetes technology still takes a lot of thought and it doesn't always stay on as well as it should. But we love the water and I'm grateful we've found ways to incorporate diabetes into summer fun. Plus, we haven't had to shave anything yet!

ASK YOUR DOCTOR

- Do you have any recommendations to help diabetes technology stay attached to skin? Do you have any samples?

- Do you have any recommended techniques for better insertion of sets or sensors?

- What can we use if infusion sets or CGM sensors irritate my child's skin?

“ Even for a very organized person, which I am not, diabetes supplies can be an enormous challenge. There are lots of boxes, tiny batteries, stuff you order every couple of weeks, and things you might buy once and never even use! ”

CHAPTER 19

Get Diabetes Organized

I still remember coming home from our first pharmacy run, just a few days after diagnosis, in 2006. We had to get syringes, insulin, a meter, testing supplies, ketone strips, and more. You probably know exactly what I mean. Six months later, we added pump supplies. A few years later, CGM stuff. Now I have all sorts of diabetes gear, most of which we still use and some that's just taking up space.

It may shock you to know that I don't consider myself a very organized person. I have found, though, that we really must keep on top of diabetes supplies. It's easy to get more Band-Aids or deodorant if we unexpectedly run out. It's a lot more difficult to get pump infusion sets.

There's a great term "diabetes overwhelmus," which was coined by the late Dr. Richard Rubin.[20] It refers, of course, to the anxiety and the amount of work that needs to be done every day just to keep up with diabetes management.

Even for a very organized person, which I am not, diabetes supplies can be an enormous challenge. There are lots of boxes, tiny batteries, stuff you order every couple of weeks, and things you might buy once and never even use! Without some kind of system, you might miss an important supply order or find yourself digging through the bottom of the junk drawer at 2:00 a.m.

Even after sixteen plus years of diabetes, I'm still surprised at just how much stuff T1D brings into our house! After all this time, I've come up with some easy ways to tame the mess and keep track of everything. Here's what works for us.

Start by taking inventory. I still do this once a year. Gather all the supplies and put everything out where you can see it. It might look like a big mess, but don't worry; you're just getting started. Group supplies together in piles or sections by use: pump stuff, CGM sensors, barrier wipes and overlays, meters, needles, etc. Make an actual list that includes everything you use, down to backup batteries and emergency glucagon.

Decide what needs to go and how you'll move it along. I always find garbage mixed in with our supplies: ripped off pieces of CGM sensor boxes, prescription labels I saved for some reason, maybe even a used sensor or infusion set. (Gross! But remember, I have a teenager.) It's easy to figure out what's trash and just throw that out.

There are some items I must keep. We don't need them anymore, but they're weirdly sentimental. I have Benny's first MedicAlert bracelet from when he was a toddler, the pretend pump we got from someone to show to his classmates, and the notebook I used in the hospital during diagnosis. We don't need those in with the current supplies, but I'm not throwing them out! I started a little "diabetes artifacts" box for those items and I store it separately. Maybe we'll put it in a real diabetes museum someday in the future. Even if those items just stay in the box, I'm not willing to throw them out.

What about anything we can't use but is still of value? This is tricky. Most diabetes charities don't take supplies, but some do. My go-to for this is Insulin for Life (https://iflusa.org/). They have terrific donation instructions on their site. You might find someone in your local area who can use the supplies. Ask your local social media groups or maybe at the next JDRF walk or in-person meetup.

As for expired items, the official advice is to throw them away. The truth is that you can use most diabetes supplies beyond that date. Understandably, you may not want to take a chance. If you find you regularly have expired supplies, you may want to rethink how often you order. We all like a stockpile, but if you will not use what you have, is it worth it?

Decide what you need at home and on the go. We have four landing spaces for diabetes supplies: Benny's backpack, kitchen drawer, laundry room shelf, and school. From there, I organize each space a bit more.

The backpack is the bane of my existence. I love purses and bags and am always on the hunt for the ones with great compartments, dividers, and anything that helps me stay neat and organized when I travel. Benny just wants a big open bag and seems to love throwing in as much as possible. As you can imagine, we have had many conversations! The compromise is bags within the bag. He uses a large zippy bag that then goes into the backpack. Within the zippy bag are smaller pouches which hold a few days' supply of everything he'd need. And garbage. I guarantee you that right now that bag is holding diabetes garbage that he just hasn't tossed yet. Again, gross, I know.

We also throw an insulin pen and a few pen needles into his bag. That way, if there's any kind of pump issue, he can inject. If the pump cartridge is empty, he can pull the insulin out of the pen and use that in the pump. I write the "no good" date on the pen and when that day rolls around, we pull all the insulin out of the pen and use it in his pump. Please note: once you suck the insulin out of the pen with the pump cartridge needle, you can no longer use the pen to inject. Air can get in and mess with the dosing.

The kitchen drawer holds a couple of weeks' worth of stuff. This is where Benny will go when he needs to change his infusion set or refill his cartridge at home. This drawer includes a great tray I got from T1D3DGear. They make all sorts of storage stuff that's personalized for your type of pump or CGM supplies.

The laundry room shelf is where I put the big boxes of pump and CGM supplies we get every three months in the mail. It also holds supplies we need but don't use as often (i.e., test strips and the backup meter). We need those a lot less often since starting CGM, but we want to keep them on hand.

Our supply at school has changed a lot over the years. For preschool and elementary school, we tried to duplicate almost everything we could. I would check just about every month to make sure they had what was needed. As Benny got older, he carried more in his backpack, but we also left supplies in the nurse's office. It's Benny's responsibility to make sure the backup stuff is there.

I get asked a lot about what Benny has used to carry what he needs. These days, as I've said, it's a backpack, but that's changed through the years. For preschool, Benny carried a little Dopp kit. In elementary school, Benny carried a little pouch with him. It was really a golf tee/supply bag, but it was a great fit and he liked it better than a small bag or backpack. Since middle school, he's carried a backpack. Most of his friends do too; everyone has electronics or other stuff they take with them these days, so that's easy.

We didn't start using Dexcom Share in earnest until the sixth grade, so I don't have experience with little kids carrying a phone around. Benny liked wearing his insulin pump in a little pouch/belt setup (similar to a SPIbelt, but a different brand). We had several versions, each with little designs like monster trucks or holiday patterns. He did eventually get a pack that held his pump and a Dexcom receiver; that was called a "double-up pouch." The receiver part was clear so you could read the number without taking it out. He played sports and wore it all summer at camp. Even though we had two, they both came home pretty gross and dirty. But it worked!

It might sound weird after all that, but I'm not a fan of little kids wearing phones. I just can't imagine my preschool or second grade son walking around all day with a phone on his hip. I can't really give you a good reason (see the previous paragraph—he wore his pump and receiver with no issues). I guess I worry about the phone breaking or just being bigger than the pump. My current iPhone is huge! A nearby backpack or string bag, or even the teacher holding the phone at recess, is good enough.

You might lose the signal for a few minutes at a time, but that's a trade-off I'd make. Plenty of kids seem to do just fine wearing their phones, so of course, that's a parental decision.

Consider clear. Finding enough space for everything at home can be tough. Whatever your system, use clear or open containers so you can see what you have. Many people love an over-the-door clear shoe organizer for this. It's a great space saver and it makes it easy for the child to get what he or she needs. Just as important, you can see what you have, so there's no reaching into a box you think has a Dexcom sensor only to find out it's empty because your child used the last one and didn't tell anyone!

Interestingly, many experts recommend we organize vertically for better focus and organization.[21] Whatever clear storage you choose, if you take items out of their original boxes, keep the lot numbers, expiration dates, and any other important info. You can take a quick photo with your phone. If you don't have clear containers or just want to use the original packaging, tape an index card to the outside and use a sharpie to keep track of what's left inside. See my comment above about the empty box frustration!

Consider using some automated help. I use my phone for lists and reminders every single day. It's an amazing diabetes personal assistant! I set reminders or alarms for ordering supplies, replenishing what we have, and for prompting me about expiration dates. If your pharmacy or mail order offers automatic ordering, consider switching over to that for as much as you can. We used to have to order Dexcom from a third party; if the order went in too late from my end, or the shipping was delayed, it was always a big problem. Switching to our local pharmacy and putting it on auto-refill is much easier. And they text me when it's ready!

Great job! Now do it again. Keeping organized takes work. I try to clean up and reorganize the kitchen drawer and our main supplies every three months, about the time we get new stuff in the mail. When Benny was younger, I'd go through his bag every

Sunday night. These days, I still check it before an overnight or a trip. Eventually, he'll be the one checking supplies, but we're not quite there yet. OK, I'm not quite there yet. My "bag check" is much more for my own peace of mind. I know he can manage, but he's not entirely on his own and this helps me feel better.

A word about insulin. I've never met anyone with so much insulin that they need to worry about organizing it. Of course, you want to keep different types separate from one another and check the temperature where you store vials or pens. Manufacturer guidelines say 36°–46°F for a year and room temperature for about a month, but recent studies (Doctors Without Borders) say it can stay just fine up to 99°F for a month.[22] That's reassuring for camp or travel, but I don't see any need to test it at home.

What about traveling?

We basically do a longer version of the three-day bag. I like to separate supplies into clear plastic bags or pouches based on how we'll use them. All insulin pump cartridges and needles go into one bag. All infusion sets go into another. I store Skin Tac and alcohol wipes in a small bag, backup meter, lancer, and lancets in another, and so on.

Benny's idea of packing is to throw everything into one bag without my cute pouches or Ziplocs. I know he's not the only teenage boy to do this, but I hate it. This is one independence step I'm not willing to let go of just yet. I still pack for our vacations because it lowers my stress level.

I have a packing list you can print out—it's in the Shop section of www.diabetes-connections.com.

The basic rule of travel is to keep your diabetes supplies with you. Keep them as carry-on for airplanes and inside the car, not the trunk. That's not just about losing your supplies; I can't tell you how many times on a long road trip we had to do an unexpected cartridge change or wanted something out of the diabetes bag. If you have the basics inside the car, you'll be fine.

Quick travel tips! Be careful about hotel refrigerators. They are notorious for freezing insulin. If you have an extended stay, test the fridge with a small cup of water. Most hotels will store medication if you don't trust the room fridge. If you're satisfied the insulin will be OK, don't forget it when you leave! My tip is to put your car keys in the fridge or near the supplies. That way, you can't leave without them. I had a listener who told me she put her shoe in the fridge with the insulin, but that's a bit extreme for me.

If you want to keep insulin colder—not just at room temperature—when you travel, I recommend the 4AllFamily cooler. It's a TSA-approved insulated thermos that can keep insulin refrigerator-cool for seventy-two hours with no power. You can also take a generic insulated thermos and pop some freezer sticks in there.

We've only had one issue with frozen insulin. We used to get our insulin via mail order, per our insurance. That meant every ninety days a big Styrofoam cooler would show up at the house. This always worked out just fine. The ice packs inside kept the insulin cool, even if it sat on the porch for a couple of hours.

One day, I got home from work and was rummaging through the fridge to figure out dinner. I opened the freezer to see the insulin cooler in the fridge. Not the insulin vials, but the big Styrofoam container. So many thoughts. First, I didn't think our freezer was that big! Second, why is the insulin here? Third, OMG! Is the insulin OK?

In my job as a radio show host, and even as a blogger, I would often get products to sample. Sometimes it was coffee from a new shop in town or a skin treatment or even shoe inserts. Not too long before this happened, it had been a new line of lower carb ice cream. The pints had arrived at the house in—you've already guessed—a big Styrofoam container, just like the one insulin comes in. Our daughter had seen the package on the porch and logically decided to put it in the freezer. She was very disappointed to learn it wasn't more mint chocolate chip!

I pulled the insulin out and called the endo. Could we still use it? How would we tell? He took us through a few questions, mostly about how it looked. It wasn't cloudy. There were no frozen bits of insulin floating in the vials. He told us he thought it would be fine and to use it. We'd know right away if it wasn't good and if there was an issue, he reassured me he'd help us get the ninety-day supply replaced.

Luckily, the insulin was fine. It wasn't in the freezer long enough to do actual damage, and I think the Styrofoam container protected it. Immense relief. I can't remember if we celebrated with ice cream, but we should have!

As long as you're organizing, here are a couple of extra steps you might want to take.

- Consider creating a medical info card or starting a small notebook you can take with you to appointments and for emergencies. It should include: all current medications, including vitamins and supplements, your doctors' contact info, your insurance info, pharmacy info, and any medication or food allergies.
- If you don't already keep a backpack or small bag of supplies, you might want to pack a go-bag for a hospital stay or an emergency trip. If you don't have enough duplicate supplies, write out what's missing (i.e., insulin from the fridge, portable charger) and leave that list taped to the outside of the bag. In an emergency, you don't want to rummage through it, guessing what you need.

Susan Weiner has an excellent book called *The Complete Diabetes Organizer* that I highly recommend. She's also the one who told me about "diabetes overwhelmus," to which I very much relate! But every time I organize our supplies, I feel a little less overwhelmed and a little more in control—for a couple of days at least!

ASK YOUR DOCTOR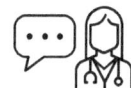

■ Can you help me reorder certain supplies or put some supplies on auto-refill?

■ Are any of my mail-order supplies now available via my pharmacy? Could that save me money?

■ What medical information would be useful to keep on hand in case of an emergency?

> **❝** It's hard to stop posting these photos, but we have to think less about the quick 'feel good' reward for our brains, and more about the impact on our children in the long run. **❞**

CHAPTER 20

Wait! Don't Share That Photo!

This chapter is hard to write. I feel very strongly about what I'm going to talk about here, but I feel like I'm swimming against the tide. You may disagree with me, but I hope you hear me out. I want to share why I'm against sharing certain images of our children, a practice that is all too common for parents in the diabetes community.

Back in 2013, I created a local Facebook group for parents of children with T1D. One of the first rules I wrote was, "We discourage sharing photos of children in distress." That's easy to agree with, right? Who would share a photo of their child on their worst day, clearly upset or ill, or in extreme anxiety or sorrow?

Turns out, lots of people do. Go to the largest diabetes parenting Facebook group you're in right now and scroll through photos. It won't take you long to find a child in a hospital bed, a child looking sad or scared, or a child who has just thrown up or is crying. People post photos of their children "in distress" all the time.

It's easy to understand why. Maybe you want to show a tough night of lows, so you share a photo of your cranky toddler with a juice box nearby. Or you post a photo of your tween in a hospital bed looking miserable because they couldn't keep fluids down and you want to warn other parents of the signs and symptoms of dehydration.

You may also think we need to show the real side of diabetes. We need to show more than the smiles when a kid gives himself a shot for the first time or decides to finally move their CGM to a new site. We need to show diabetes isn't fair. I agree with that. I am all for realism; I promise it is not sunshine and unicorns and rainbows over here.

However, to show the "real" side of diabetes, we don't need to exploit our children. Strong language, but I believe that's what's happening here. These are children, many of whom are too young to give consent to be featured, but have just as much right to their privacy as we do.

I think about how I'd feel if someone took a photo of me at my most vulnerable and posted it on Facebook or Instagram. I can imagine how I'd react if my husband took a quick picture just as I'd gotten sick or was hungover or exhausted. Even if Slade meant well ("Look how hard my wife is working," or "Isn't she an amazing trooper through this illness?"), I know I wouldn't appreciate looking my worst in an image that will be around forever.

I did a little research on this and, as you can imagine, there are a lot of articles about social media and photos. To be clear, though, there's not a lot of peer-reviewed research because this is still so new.

Dr. Kristy Goodwin is the author of *Raising Your Child in a Digital World*.[23] She has a PhD in the impact of digital technology on children's learning. She says that, right now, sharing every part of our lives has been normalized by social media. If you dial back, though, it's a desire to feel connected. Dr. Goodwin says this is one of our biological drivers as a human, and we need it to experience empathy. So the desire for those clicks and likes serves a real purpose.

"For many parents when their kids are seriously sick, they have lost all control and their world is literally spinning out of control," says Dr. Goodwin. "When parents go on social media, they have a sense of control over their life again. They can post things and choose exactly what aspects of their child's sickness that they want to post."[24]

Another article is from a pediatric hospitalist from St. Louis Children's Hospital, Dr. Shobha Bhaskar. She says: "We are all looking for support when our loved ones are not well. But when your child is running a fever or has a broken bone, please put down the camera, step away from the screen and go take care of them! I'm sure that if your child had a choice, they want to look their best too (like you do) and does not appreciate a picture of them looking tired and run down on the emergency room bed. So if you should post, keep the details and description minimal. We talk so much about patient privacy rules and rights, but what about the privacy rights of our little ones? Or do we think that they just don't have any!?"[25]

These photos are shared because we love our kids. We want to get attention and feel connected while dealing with a tough situation. Often, these are the posts that get the most likes and comments, which feels great. Lots of studies show that positive feedback in social media triggers a dopamine release in our bodies. That's the "feel-good" chemical that's also released when we eat delicious food or have a great social interaction.

The Cleveland Clinic says: "As humans, our brains are hard-wired to seek out behaviors that release dopamine in our reward system. When you're doing something pleasurable, your brain releases a large amount of dopamine. You feel good and you seek more of that feeling. This is why junk food and sugar are so addictive. They trigger the release of a large amount of dopamine into your brain, which gives you the feeling that you're on top of the world and you want to repeat that experience."[26]

Any wonder why we seek to post more photos that give us the greatest rewards? It's hard to stop, but we have to think less about the rewards for our brains, and more about the impact on our children. In my group, I try to discourage posting these photos at all. Here's one of the rules:

Please think twice about any pictures you post of your children, especially those of your child in distress. This includes hospital pictures, pictures during illness, etc. You have our support and sympathy already; your child has his or her own right to privacy and may not appreciate being pictured online in such a manner. These pictures aren't banned. But take a moment to think about why you might want to post something like that.

You'll note that I don't actually ban these photos outright. Why not? After all, I just got on my high horse and told you how terrible they were! I don't ban them because I want to have this conversation. I want people to think about why they're posting and whether they really want to. An outright ban might create a more closed-minded atmosphere. So far, it's been a great conversation starter.

Whenever anybody posts this kind of photo, I usually send them a very gentle, private message, reiterating what I already talked about here. The message is: We support you; we love you; we're so sorry your child is hurting. But why are you posting that picture? Can you please think about your child's privacy?

Sometimes I wait, because if the child is ill, there's no reason for the parents to hear from me when they're in the hospital. I have no desire to message a parent whose child is in a critical situation only to ask that they check a photo on Facebook. But once I reach out, they usually understand. I don't remember one parent who got upset with me for asking them to think about this issue.

I practice what I preach, even when I want to post more. Benny had knee surgery twice in the last two years. You bet I took pictures. We took funny pictures when they shaved his leg. I took a picture of his pump in the hospital gown pocket. I took pictures of him giving a thumbs up going into surgery and a picture of him coming out and bundled in so many blankets we couldn't see him!

He was fine, just cold coming out of the anesthesia. Most of those are not pictures he'd want me to post, but he wanted to see them later on.

Benny also had a scary accident when he was eight years old, which sent us to an unfamiliar ER. Once we knew he was going to be OK, I took a few photos. I'm glad I did. It allowed me to share information and better communicate with my mom and my sister, and I showed them to Benny later on. But I've never posted them anywhere.

That's a good example of privacy in a different way. If you're a longtime listener of the podcast, you may think, "I've never heard about this scary accident! What happened to Benny?" I know it seems like I lay everything out in these books and on the show, but I don't share everything. I work hard to protect the privacy of my kids and my family in ways that make sense to me. Not every story needs to be made public. That one had nothing to do with diabetes and he's absolutely fine now.

In situations where I want to connect and share photos, I try to get a little creative. During the knee surgery, I posted a photo of hospital equipment without him in the shot. Several years ago, after a night of infusion set changes and a bunch of lows, I took a picture of his bedside table. It was covered with juice boxes and test strips and diabetes tech trash; it looked like a war zone. That conveyed the difficulty of type 1 diabetes without pulling a lousy-feeling kid into the shot.

I think one reason I notice these types of photos is because I didn't have social media until my youngest child was close to kindergarten age. I joined Twitter and Facebook in 2008 and it would be a few years before influencer-type photos of children and even closed groups would become part of the landscape.

When Benny was diagnosed in 2006, we didn't carry cameras everywhere because very few phones had that feature! It's wild to think how much technology has changed. I wish I had those photos, though. It was a sad day, but there were many funny and touching moments as well. I'd like to see him being so brave and getting his first shot, his sister hugging him, and meeting our endo for the first time. I have all of those snapshots in my head, but having the actual pictures would be nice.

This next matter is also a parenting decision, not just a diabetes one. My daughter has never had an active social media account. She's asked us, since age thirteen or fourteen, to please not share photos of her unless she's OK'd them. Unless they're really weird or embarrassing, she's almost always OK with what I put out there, but these conversations with her have also made me consider carefully what and where I post. Some of my friends have told me they feel their kids' images belong to the parent and they can share whenever and wherever they want. That may be legally true, but it doesn't feel right to me. If a child asks you to stop sharing, I think that's an important expression of autonomy and can be the start of a great conversation.

I asked about this type of oversharing on social media, curious about what others in the diabetes community thought. The feedback was fascinating. Almost every adult with diabetes asked me to please tell parents not to post pictures of their children. They either felt their parents had overdone it or they felt it put the person with diabetes in a powerless position, regardless of age.

Many parents and some advocates have said not sharing these images would hurt fundraising efforts. I don't buy it. We've been fundraising for JDRF and some other causes for fifteen years. We might have raised close to $100,000. I have never once shared a photo of Benny in distress to raise money. Has he been in distress? You bet. Have I written and talked about it? Sure. But we have found creative ways to show our lives with T1D. I know many, many other people who have raised a lot more money than us, who have never posted a sick-day photo of their child.

I also heard from people concerned about what this could do for education, especially around diabetic ketoacidosis (DKA) at diagnosis. The most dangerous time to be type 1 is before anybody knows that you are; DKA can be deadly. Right now, about 46 percent of patients with type 1 are in diabetes ketoacidosis at the time of diagnosis in the United States.[27] There are several campaigns to get medical professionals to recognize diabetes earlier. Don't we need to show what can happen?

Yes. However, the most impactful photo I ever saw around DKA wasn't anyone's face. It was a pair of shoes.

Beyond Type 1 did a wonderful bit of photojournalism a few years ago called "Previously Healthy." It featured the story of a toddler, Reegan Oxendine, who was misdiagnosed again and again. Finally, she was hospitalized, but it was too late. It's a terrible and sad story. Beyond Type 1 told it with care and dignity and the photo they ran with it was Reegan's mother's hands, holding the toddler's tiny shoes.[28] It's incredibly powerful, but it's not exploitive.

Most of us aren't photojournalists and we don't have to worry about our images being shared worldwide. But we all must be aware that the internet is public and forever. That quick shot of my sad looking five-year-old isn't going anywhere; it's very possible that child will find it when he's older. Even if you've posted in a closed Facebook group, nothing is truly private. The minute you post, somebody else can screenshot it, save it, or forward it; you have no idea where it might go.

I guess what I'm asking is: take a moment to think, 'Why am I doing this? What do I need right now?' If it's support and sympathy, I promise it's out there. If it's showing the "real" side of diabetes, I promise there's a way to show that without exploiting your child. Take a few extra minutes to decide why you're sharing that photo and remember that you can't take it back once it's out there. If it feels right and you decide to share, go for it. The diabetes community will offer empathy and understanding whenever you need it.

> ❝ 'Motherhood is juggling? I'm the mom of a kid with type 1. I can juggle flaming chainsaws!' I have bad news for you. You really can't. At least not by yourself. ❞

CHAPTER 21

Juggling Flaming Chainsaws—a Bit about Self-Care

D o you ever do a "word of the year?" I don't make resolutions anymore, but I love the idea of selecting a word. It's a great way to set the tone you want for the year, refer to it later on, and to see what you were thinking even years later.

So far, I've had "finish," "opportunity," and "forge." For 2022, my word was "calibrate."

That has nothing to do with CGMs! Dictionary.com's definition of calibrate is: "to determine, check, or rectify the graduation of (any instrument giving quantitative measurements)." In this case, I'm the instrument. I want to check in with myself throughout the year and make sure I'm as balanced as I can be.

For me, balance isn't about perfectly even scales (even though I am a Libra). Balance means prioritizing what's important at the moment, meeting long-term goals, and taking breaks to have some fun and pay attention to myself. I work. I have children and a husband and I like to play golf. I love to read, see friends, and walk my dog. I'm always starting a new side project. I like to be busy, but I also need to make sure I'm not over-committed.

Motherhood is juggling even without diabetes, but you have to take care of the juggler, or all those balls will come crashing down. I know what you're thinking, "I will just keep juggling even if those balls catch on fire. I'm the mom of a kid with type 1. I can juggle flaming chainsaws!"

I have bad news for you. You really can't. At least not by yourself. I know this because I tried.

I want to share a story about myself. It's hard to write about this because I usually keep the focus on our diabetes stories. This is more about my struggles with sleep and health.

Bit of a trigger warning in this part of the chapter: illness and hospitalization.

In 2012, I almost died. I wish that was an exaggeration or me just being dramatic. But it's true. I spent two weeks in the hospital and for a few days, they weren't sure I was going to make it home. What I learned made me fiercely protective of my sleep and my health. In our society, and in the diabetes community, that sentence alone would probably make me "the worst" kind of mom.

I was working at my radio job, the one I'd had since just after my daughter was born. I got to work at 4:00 a.m. each day, which meant leaving my house by 3:15 a.m. Morning radio is a horrible schedule, but when my children were tiny, it wasn't so bad. We all went to bed by 7:30 p.m. I was lucky to have great childcare, so if I needed more sleep during the day, I could take a quick nap and then go get the kids.

During this time, my husband owned and operated a restaurant, so he would take care of the kids in the morning, but he often wouldn't come home until close to midnight. When Benny was diagnosed, we were the rare parents who didn't struggle with middle-of-the-night checks, because one of us was awake at 12:00 a.m. and the other was up at 3:00 a.m.

As the children got older, though, my schedule became a problem. Elementary school activities rarely end in time for a 7:30 p.m. bedtime and, as Lea started middle school, we often weren't getting to bed before 9:00 p.m. I started getting about four or five hours of sleep a night; something quick naps couldn't fix.

In early 2012, I got very sick. I was suddenly nauseous and exhausted. Since I was always tired, I chalked it up to my schedule. One morning, though, I knew I needed to leave. I made it through my last "live-read" commercial (I didn't want the sales guys to make up the loss, something my coworkers and I still laugh about) and then threw up in the bathroom. I saw my doctor the next day. To my shock, he referred me to a liver specialist! I was having an extremely rare allergic reaction to some medication and it was shutting down my liver.

There was no treatment other than stopping the medication and resting. I slept, no joke, twenty hours a day for the next two weeks. I saved up all my energy to put the kids to bed; reading to them and tucking them in was pretty much the only thing I did during that time. Finally, almost a full month later, I went back to work.

I wish that was the end of the story. Instead, just a couple of weeks later, I was having similar, but even more severe, symptoms. My liver checked out fine. No one could figure out what was wrong. I was hospitalized and they ran test after test. I remember little after being admitted; apparently, they thought I might have an infectious disease, but treatments didn't work. I needed two blood transfusions and the doctors were telling my husband they were getting worried.

Finally, about five days later, I was diagnosed with an autoimmune disease. Thankfully, the treatment worked, but I had a long road of recovery ahead of me. I spent another month at home.

What I have can be tricky. It can flare up frequently, be very well controlled with just a little trouble once or twice a year, or it can go into remission entirely. I was lucky to manage very well for about five years and then gradually come off all medication. I'm considered in remission and have been for about four years now.

My doctor says we'll never really know why my body reacted the way it did, but he suspects it was because I was getting a ridiculously low amount of sleep. Now you know why I share this story.

When your child has diabetes, it can seem like the only logical thing to do is never sleep again. If you hang out in some social media groups, this is reinforced repeatedly. It's become part of our diabetes mom culture; you've seen the posts with #TeamNoSleep and #SendCoffee. I'm here to tell you, it's not sustainable. And it's not required.

I don't mean you should ignore CGM alarms or never check your child overnight. I want you to think about how we can use the tools we have to find ways to get more sleep. That might mean turning the Dexcom high alarm to 250 for a night or two. Or turning the high alarm off entirely once you've already treated for the night.

If your partner or spouse is able to help overnight but doesn't, please have an honest conversation with them. I often think my husband knows exactly what I want him to do, but after twenty-five years together, he's still a terrible mind reader. You might need to ask them to take over two nights a week. Stick to that and sleep in another room and turn off your alarms, if that's what it takes.

If you're on your own with this, I have the utmost respect for what you're going through, and I can't pretend there are easy answers. We had no family nearby, so we trained lots of friends and used caregivers when we wanted a night away. Sitters can become expensive, so lean on your local community. Maybe there's another D-Mom who will host your child for a sleepover. You can return the favor and you both can get some rest.

I want to be clear that I'm not judging anyone who has to stay awake with a child; that's just part of being a parent. I don't know anyone with children who gets as much sleep as my friends without kids! What I've been talking about here is the culture, which seems to make a lack of sleep a badge of honor or a necessity. It's troubling to me that anyone would assign a moral value to sleeplessness or indicate you're a better mom if you get less sleep.

I am reluctant to give more specific advice about sleep here, as it brings me into medical-type territory. But I would urge you to talk to your care team. I know the fear that keeps us awake and I'm telling you, it's unfounded. The most dangerous time for a person with type 1 diabetes is before they're diagnosed, when no one realizes they have diabetes, which can lead to DKA. There is a fear in our community that our children are one overnight low or high blood sugar away from an emergency. That's just not the case.

Besides sleep issues, we carry the regular stress of diabetes management. While there are issues specific to your child's age and stage of T1D diagnosis, there are questions we all carry around. Am I doing enough? Am I doing too much? Will this dosing be correct for this meal or this activity? Is my child ready to manage this bit of diabetes independently?

For many of us, those questions start to fade into the background as diabetes becomes more and more routine. But if you find you just can't let down your guard, even for an hour, I'd encourage you to talk to your doctor or even your child's endo. I know many parents who've been helped by counseling and even medication when necessary. Of course, that's between you and your health care provider, but therapy can be a wonderful tool. I wish mental health was addressed immediately after a diabetes diagnosis—for the person with diabetes and for family members.

I'm happy to share that I've spoken to a therapist for the last couple of years. When my daughter went to college, I found that I needed some help to figure out how I felt about this new phase of life. It's been wonderful, especially during the stress of COVID. I didn't seek her out because of diabetes, but of course it comes up.

I still lean heavily on my community of diabetes moms. Here's a good example of when I really needed some love and support from people who get it.

When I talked about Benny's trip to Israel, I mentioned that part of the way I managed remote monitoring when he was so far away was by limiting the number of times a day I looked at his numbers. I would look every morning when I woke up, and about an hour before I went to bed. This was a plan I worked out with my therapist, and it kept me from staring at the Dexcom all day. It worked well for me, but it was still a stressful month.

During the time of the trip, I attended the annual Friends for Life Conference, held every summer at a Disney resort conference center. At one meetup of moms, everyone jokingly decided to put their phones on the table. "No matter what the number is, show us your kid's Dexcom graph!"

The numbers were all over the place and the dozen or so moms at the food court table shared a laugh and talked about how great it was to be together. They noticed I wasn't looking at Benny's numbers. "It's not time," I explained.

They gently pushed me to join in. I agreed, telling myself it was just one day off my routine. When would I have the chance to be with a dozen diabetes moms again? I said OK, opened the Dexcom Follow app, and threw my phone in the pile.

Of course, Benny's blood sugar was 77 with an arrow going straight down. I burst into tears.

Was he fine? Of course. He wasn't alone; he was already two weeks into his trip and had treated a bunch of lower numbers with no issues. We only had a handful of urgent low alarms the whole time he was away, and this wouldn't become one of those times.

This was just about me. I think because I was finally surrounded by people who understood, I could let go. My close friends listened when I talked about my concerns, but I think unless you live with type 1 in your family, you really can't understand. I was happy to let Benny go on this once-in-a-lifetime trip. But I was scared as well. All of that came pouring out in the food court at the Coronado Springs Resort.

I didn't realize until after it happened, but I needed to let that stress out. I needed that cry. After I shared with that group of women who truly understood my concerns, I felt lighter. I was still worried, of course, but the feeling was different. Other moms shared about their experiences letting T1D kids travel abroad and how their young adults moved far away. The moms of younger kids talked about how great it was to hear these stories of children with T1D becoming independent.

As I've said many times before, a terrific way to start your child on that road is with diabetes camp. Another reason camp is great, though, is because it allows parents to have a break. As moms, we need more times in our lives when we can be a little selfish. Diabetes camp can be the one week in the year when you let it all go. If your child hasn't been to camp yet, you might feel very apprehensive, but it really is one of the safest places for them. And it gives you a chance to recharge and relax.

It's not always possible to carve out time for yourself. But I hope you think about calibrating your busy life now and then. Check in with yourself. Step back and see what you need. And if you can't stop juggling right now, recognize it's OK to ask for help.

ASK YOUR DOCTOR

■ Are there any local babysitting services that are known to be helpful for T1D families?

■ Can you give us some advice to help our overnights be more restful? How can I keep my child safe and still get some sleep?

■ How can I better train more caregivers? Does your office offer any additional education?

❝ There's no multiverse situation where I become the perfect diabetes mom. And even with enough do-overs, would I want to? ❞

CHAPTER 22

What's Next?

"**M**om, I'm fine."
That could be the title of every T1D child's autobiography. You know what I mean. When you text and remind them to bolus, or yell upstairs that they need to change a sensor, that's their go-to response.

"Mom, I've got it. It's fine."

As I look ahead to the very near future when Benny will go off to college and move on, I have to remind myself that it really is fine. I've always said we don't expect perfection with diabetes, and we've certainly never modeled or taught it. So why would I imagine it will suddenly happen in this next phase of life? Mistakes keep happening, we keep learning, and Benny continues to be safe and happy.

Recently, he was going out with friends and was in a bit of a hurry to get ready. He asked me to fill an insulin cartridge for him while he jumped into the shower. I was happy to help, so I filled the cartridge and left it on the kitchen counter for him. I sat back down on the couch and a few minutes later, I heard him bustling around in the kitchen. Then he left.

About ten minutes after he departed, I noticed the cartridge was still on the counter. Maybe it was the old one? He usually throws the trash away when he does changes like this, so I texted him.

He'd completely forgotten to take it with him. While he wasn't out of insulin yet, they were going out to eat and to the movies, so he'd need that new cartridge. He texted me he was on his way back.

When he got home, he was laughing. He has a few other friends with type 1 and he was hanging out with one of them that night. "Mom, Parker forgot his insulin too. We both had to leave to come home and get it."

Mothers of teens, a reminder: Your child is not alone in their forgetfulness.

We were in Boston for a college visit earlier this year. Benny had his bag as always while we toured during the day. We rested up at our hotel and decided on an Italian restaurant for dinner. We were told it was only about a ten-minute walk, so Benny left his stuff at the hotel. As I've explained, he uses the Tandem/Dexcom combo so no external controller is needed. He threw a roll of glucose tabs in his pocket, and we were off.

Three minutes into our walk, he skimmed his arm along a fence and ripped out the Dexcom. *Sigh.* I told him to put the transmitter into his pocket so we wouldn't lose it and to look at his number while he still had one. That way, at least we'd have a baseline going into dinner. He was 76 with a diagonal arrow down, indicating his BG was dropping slowly. He felt fine, so he chomped a few tabs and we kept walking.

We had a wonderful dinner, walked all over Cambridge, and replaced the Dexcom sensor back at the hotel about two and a half hours later. Was it ideal? Of course not. We didn't have a meter with us and for that short period of time, we didn't know what his blood sugar was. That would have made me very nervous when he was younger and newly diagnosed. However, after all this time, we've learned that diabetes is rarely an emergency and not knowing every number, every second, is OK. I think what terrified me is how much he ate! Seventeen-year-old appetites are no joke!

When your youngest child is about to graduate high school, I think it inspires a lot of introspection and emotions. Whether they plan to leave for college or stay close by, it represents the end of an era. I'm having a bit of trouble writing these words, but it represents the end of childhood. That's significant no matter what your family's situation, but, as usual, having a child with diabetes adds another layer.

I worry if we've done enough. My time teaching Benny about T1D is almost over. Have we taught him enough? Should I have been stricter about numbers? Should I have concentrated more on trying to be maybe a little bit perfect?

I had an interesting conversation about this with my husband. I was talking about both kids, how they're both almost adults and that I wonder if we should have done anything differently. He looked at it another way. His take was that no matter what we do, we'll never know what would have been. No matter the method, we'd always wonder about the alternative. We've done our best. We love our children and we can't worry about what might have been.

Telling me not to worry is never effective, but he made sense. There's no multiverse situation where I become the perfect diabetes mom. And even with enough do-overs, would I want to?

Benny spent this past summer at his non-diabetes sleepaway camp. It was his longest time away from home yet, eight weeks as a Counselor in Training (CIT). He's wanted to be a CIT at this camp since the minute he got there at age eight. He talked about it after camp every summer and around age eleven or twelve, he asked me what he had to do to make it happen.

"That's not up to me," I said. "You apply to the camp, and they decide if you're a good candidate."

"No, I mean with diabetes," he explained. "What do I have to do to make you let me go?"

It hadn't occurred to me he thought there was some kind of diabetes test or hurdle he had to pass. He knew this role had more responsibility and he recognized we were giving him a chance every summer to show he was up to the challenge.

"Just keep doing what you're doing, kiddo," I said. "As long as you're safe and happy and the camp is OK with how we're managing, there's nothing else you need to worry about."

He was surprised and excited. We had a few years to go, but I was happy to reassure him that this experience wasn't out of reach. And now he's done it. As we look forward to college and beyond, I'm trying to reassure myself that as long as he's safe and happy, it will continue to be OK.

I took some solace in a study I read this year. It was all about transitioning older teenagers from pediatric to adult endocrinologists. We're lucky that Dr. V will keep seeing Benny at least through college, but the study shined some light on what these kids are thinking and what support they want.

Besides worrying that their adult doctors wouldn't be as invested in them and about logistics of managing their own health insurance and supplies, the teens talked about independence. They were very aware and concerned about their changing relationship with their parents. Some wanted to take on more responsibility in diabetes management, but "experienced excessive supervision by parents."[29]

Ouch! That phrase is a bit harsh, but it makes an important point. As much as we hate it, one of our important jobs as parents is to give our children the tools to be independent and then to be brave enough to let them use those tools. I believe in that deeply. Our job is to let go, but boy, do I struggle with it!

We have decisions to make over the next year. Will I remote monitor in college? Right now, I'm leaning toward no. Will I still help with ordering supplies and making sure Benny has what he needs? Most likely.

In my talk with Benny about Israel, I asked him what he wanted from us going forward. That resulted in the "customer support" decision. But he said something else to me that resonated and has influenced how I talk to him about diabetes.

"You have done great. You have done wonderful. And if you want to get a bit more naggy, you can get a bit more naggy. It's not going to change anything."

I'm going to translate some Benny-speak here. I think what he really means is: 'Mom, I've learned so much from you and dad and Dr. V. But at this point, I'm taking over my diabetes management. You can nag if you want, but it's up to me now.'

Let's go back to the photo I mentioned in the introduction, of that little boy jumping off the boat. Remember, he's got his life vest on. We've taught him how to swim. Am I worried? Of course! But living life on your mom's lap on the boat after you've got the skills and tools you need to leap off is no fun.

We've helped him fly. Now it's time to watch him soar.

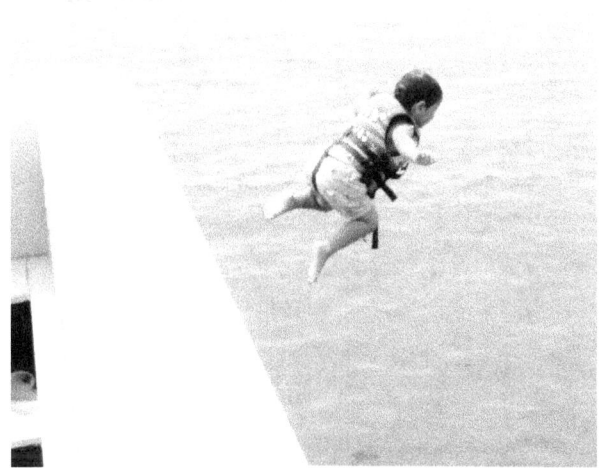

Acknowledgments

I have loved writing these books. Thank you to everyone who has read *The World's Worst Diabetes Mom* and reached out. I've tried to respond to every comment, every email, and every DM. They all mean the world to me.

Thank you to my podcast audience, guests, and especially the Diabetes Connections Facebook group. You are always ready to answer my questions, give feedback, and keep me going in the right direction.

I'm very grateful to Anna Sabino, MSW, CDCES of Finding Smiles Coaching, for reading an early version of this book. Anna asked questions and pushed me to think about some subjects in a way that helped me clarify the writing and pinpoint exactly what I wanted to say. Thank you to Moira McCarthy for allowing me to share her words within this book and for all of her advice along the way. I could not ask for a better D-Mom mentor and friend.

Our health-care team continues to be a tireless resource, and I appreciate their willingness to let me share our stories. Thank you especially to Dr. Mark Vanderwel; Linnet Steinman, CDCES, MSN, RN; Justin Thomas; and the staffs of Camp Kudos and Camp Morris. I also can't say enough about the staff at URJ Camp Coleman, especially Karen Greenspan and Neri Thompson, and NFTY in Israel.

Thank you to the staff at SPARK Publications. Fabi Preslar's confidence and steady hand once again guided me. Larry Preslar's enthusiastic and patient responses to all of my graphic and design questions kept me engaged in the part of the process I find quite difficult. I adore the changes we made to the cover image!

To my sister, Melissa, for her incredible encouragement in real life and online. She is quick to retweet or share my posts and give enthusiastic feedback. Plus, I can count on her to tell me when something stinks. Thanks, sis! As always, my parents are a source of unwavering support. My mother's "life" advice always seems to work out for diabetes too. What a gift to have Steve and Arlene in my corner!

Thank you to Lea for being willing to share more of herself here and to Benny for allowing me to tell so many stories. I'm incredibly proud that you both are generous in ways that will help other families. I'm humbled and grateful that you trust me to only share what you've approved.

To Slade, for listening to my fears about how the first book would be received and whether I was going too far with my opinions in this one. For bringing me dinner when I'm on deadline and for supplying all the coffee. Our family's adventures are about to look a lot different as the kids move on. Looking forward to the next chapter with you!

About the Author

Stacey Simms hosts the long-running and award-winning podcast "Diabetes Connections." Her previous book *The World's Worst Diabetes Mom* won several awards, including Best New Nonfiction from American BookFest. Stacey's son was diagnosed with type 1 diabetes in 2006, one month before he turned two years old, and Stacey started blogging about her family's experience with T1D a few weeks later. For more than a decade, she hosted "Charlotte's Morning News" on WBT-AM, the city's top-rated morning radio news show. Stacey has been named to *Diabetes Forecast* magazine's People to Know, the *Charlotte Business Journal's* 40 Under 40, and *Mecklenburg Times'* 50 Most Influential Women. She lives near Charlotte, North Carolina, with her husband, their two children, and their dog, Freckles.

CONNECT WITH STACEY ONLINE

🌐 diabetes-connections.com

🌐 staceysimms.com

⬤ diabetesconnections

⬤ staceysimms

⬤ staceysimms

Endnotes

1 Stacey Simms, "Trick or Treat," November 1, 2007, https://staceysimms.com/trick-or-treat-2/.

2 Manuel (Manny) Hernandez, "Percentage of Time Spent by People with Diabetes with a Medical Professional in a Year," October 1, 2015, https://www.mannyhernandez.co/blog/2015/10/of-time-spent-by-people-with-diabetes-with-a-medical-professional-in-a-year.

3 Stacey Simms, "You Deserve a Medal," June 28, 2012, https://staceysimms.com/medalist/.

4 Joslin Diabetes, "Honoring Joslin's Heroes," Medalist Program & Study, accessed June 29, 2022, https://www.joslin.org/research/our-research/medalist-program-study.

5 Stacey Simms, "Party Like a Doctor," April 2, 2013, https://staceysimms.com/party-like-a-doctor/.

6 American Diabetes Association, "The History of a Wonderful Thing We Call Insulin," July 1, 2019, https://www.diabetes.org/blog/history-wonderful-thing-we-call-insulin#:~:text=In%201910%2C%20Sir%20Edward%20Albert,insula%2C%20meaning%20%E2%80%9Cisland.%E2%80%9D.

7 Stephen R. Covey, *The 7 Habits of Highly Effective People,* (New York: Simon & Schuster, 2020).

8 Stacey Simms, "Interview: Artificial Pancreas," April 16, 2013, https://staceysimms.com/interview-artificial-pancreas/.

9 Stacey Simms, "Dexcom First Impressions," January 15, 2014, https://staceysimms.com/dexcom-first-impressions/.

10 Stacey Simms, "Find My Dexcom," January 9, 2014, https://staceysimms.com/find-my-dexcom/.

11 Lina Alkhaled et al., "1381-P: Psychological Characteristics of Caregivers Choosing Continuous Glucose Monitoring (CGM) for Their Children with Type 1 Diabetes (T1D)," *Diabetes 68, Supplement_1 (2019)* 1381–P. https://doi.org/10.2337/db19-1381-P.

12 Manuela Sinisterra et al., "Young Children with Type 1 Diabetes: Sleep, Health-Related Quality of Life, and Continuous Glucose Monitor Use," Diabetes Technology & Therapeutics 22, no. 8 (2020):639-642. https://www.ncbi.nlm.nih.gov/pmc/articles/PMC7406998/.

13 Sarah Tackett, "Celebrating 2 Years of the T1D Exchange Registry," T1D Exchange, accessed July 27, 2022, https://t1dexchange.org/celebrating-2-years-of-the-t1d-exchange-registry/.

14 Stacey Simms, "The Pump & the Potty," August 8, 2007, https://staceysimms.com/the-pump-the-po/.

15 Steven Edelman, "The Un-Tethered Regimen," Children with Diabetes, Diabetes Technology & Therapeutics 22, no. 8 (2020) accessed July 27, 2022, https://childrenwithdiabetes.com/un-tethered-regimen/#:~:text=Steven%20Edelman%20(2004)&text=The%20un%2Dtethered%20regimen%20refers,flexible%20and%20user%20friendly%20manner.

16 Moira McCarthy, "The a1C: Golden Trophy or Scarlet Number? Time to Take Away the Shame," Despite Diabetes, December 28, 2011, http://www.despitediabetes.com/the-a1c-golden-trophy-or-scarlet-number-time-to-take-away-the-shame/.

17 Megan Molteni, "Top Privacy Researchers Urge the Healthcare Industry to Safeguard Patient Data," STAT, Health Tech, May 24, 2022, https://www.statnews.com/2022/05/24/health-data-privacy-patients-records/?utm_content=buffer4766d&utm_medium=social&utm_source=twitter&utm_campaign=twitter_organic.

18 Doctors Without Borders, "MSF Study Shows Some Insulin Can Be Stored at Warmer Temperatures," February 3, 2021, https://www.doctorswithoutborders.org/latest/msf-study-shows-some-insulin-can-be-stored-warmer-temperatures.

19 Moira McCarthy, *Raising Teens with Diabetes: A Survival Guide for Parents,* (Spry Publishing LLC, 2013).

20 Richard R. Rubin, "Diabetes and Quality of Life," *Diabetes Spectrum* 13, no. 1 (2000): 21, accessed July 8, 2022, https://link.gale.com/apps/doc/A61370256/AONE?u=anon~dd85aaa7&sid=googleScholar&xid=7a1d3690.

21 Stacey Simms "Get Diabetes Organized! Help & Advice for the New Year," January 2, 2018, in Diabetes Connections, guest Susan Weiner, podcast, audio, 46:51, https://diabetes-connections.com/get-diabetes-organized-help-advice-for-the-new-year/.

22 Doctors Without Borders, "MSF Study Shows Some Insulin Can Be Stored at Warmer Temperatures," February 3, 2021, https://www.doctorswithoutborders.org/latest/msf-study-shows-some-insulin-can-be-stored-warmer-temperatures.

23 Kristy Goodwin, *Raising Your Child in a Digital World: What You Need to Know!,* (Finch Publishing, 2016).

24 Joshua Barrie, "Doctor Says Parents Posting Photos of Their Sick Children Is 'Self Promotion,'" Mirror, March 10, 2018, https://www.mirror.co.uk/lifestyle/family/doctor-says-parents-posting-photos-12163389?fbclid=IwAR14DzCAk2d2Z371mAnQvm2Kz6EWZUBVUsNlop8S1EIWCNF43xqfxhDkOW4.

25 Shobha Bhaskar, "Mom, Please Don't Post That!" Children's MD, August 13, 2015, https://childrensmd.org/browse-by-age-group/toddler-pre-school/mom-please-dont-post/.

26 Cleveland Clinic, "Dopamine," accessed July 8, 2022, https://my.clevelandclinic.org/health/articles/22581-dopamine.

27 Beyond Type 1, "Our Warning Signs Awareness Campaign," accessed July 22, 2022, https://beyondtype1.org/dkacampaign/.

28 Michelle Boise, "Previously Healthy," Beyond Type 1, accessed July 31, 2022, https://beyondtype1.org/?s=previously+healthy.

29 Erin T. Welsh, "Novel Programs Needed to Improve Transition from Pediatric to Adult Diabetes Care," Endocrine Today, April 4, 2022, https://www.healio.com/news/endocrinology/20220401/novel-programs-needed-to-improve-transition-from-pediatric-to-adult-diabetes-care.

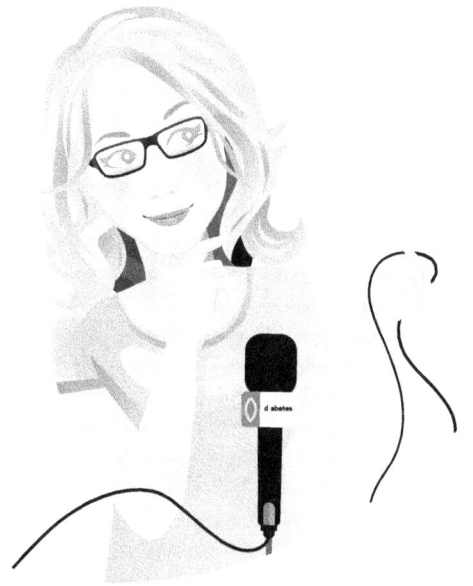

diabetes-connections.com

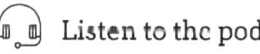 Listen to the podcast.

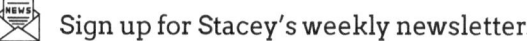 Sign up for Stacey's weekly newsletter.

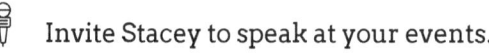 Invite Stacey to speak at your events.

www.ingramcontent.com/pod-product-compliance
Lightning Source LLC
Chambersburg PA
CBHW061146120626
46546CB00005B/1949